Plastic Surgery

PLASTIC SURGERY

The Kindest Cut

John Camp

HENRY HOLT AND COMPANY / New York

For Susan

Copyright © 1989 by John Camp
All rights reserved, including the right to reproduce this
book or portions thereof in any form.
Published by Henry Holt and Company, Inc.,
115 West 18th Street, New York, New York 10011.
Published in Canada by Fitzhenry & Whiteside Limited,
195 Allstate Parkway, Markham, Ontario L3R 4T8.

Library of Congress Cataloging-in-Publication Data
Camp, John.
Plastic surgery : the kindest cut / John Camp.—1st ed.
p.   cm.
Includes index.
ISBN 0-8050-0897-7
1. Surgery, Plastic—Popular works.   I. Title.
RD119.C35   1989
617′.95—dc19   88-13721
CIP

Henry Holt books are available at special discounts
for bulk purchases for sales promotions, premiums,
fund-raising, or educational use. Special editions
or book excerpts can also be created to specification.

For details, contact:

Special Sales Director
Henry Holt and Company, Inc.
115 West 18th Street
New York, New York 10011

First Edition

Designed by Paula R. Szafranski
Printed in the United States of America
1   3   5   7   9   10   8   6   4   2

Contents

Introduction

BEAUTY IS important.

It may be critical.

And somewhere, at the bottom of the mind, everybody knows it.

A few minutes after six o'clock on a bleak winter morning, a patient got out of a car near the hospital's front entrance. She said, "Okay, see ya," into the open door, slammed it, and rapped on the car's roof with her knuckles. She looked back once as the car crept away between the streetlights.

The patient carried a purse and a navy-blue nylon athletic bag with an airline insignia on the side. She walked firmly along the sidewalk between strips of dirty meltdown snow, her head bent against the stinging ice crystals and bits of scrap paper and other late-winter debris blown along the street by a vicious northwest wind.

The hospital was small and homely. Built of red brick, it snuggled on a side street in an aging neighborhood, surrounded by clapboard houses with black-screened porches and small lawns.

Inside the hospital doors, the patient, who had grown up in snow country, automatically stamped her feet on the rubber mat before she walked up the stairs to the information desk. The desk clerk, yawning, directed the patient to the elevators that would take her to the operating suite.

The patient was a dark-eyed, dark-haired young woman, with olive skin and strong white teeth. In another time, in another culture—a culture of the eastern Mediterranean, perhaps—she would have been a beauty. In America, in the 1980s, she was not. Not quite.

That would change over the next two hours. In a delicate, artful operation, a plastic surgeon would alter the entire aspect of her face, and, quite possibly, her life.

Most Americans like to believe that success in life derives from merit and hard work. It offends us, somehow, that success should commonly depend on matters of physical appearance.

Whatever exceptions might be cited, there are mountains of evidence that appearance is a crucial matter. It always has been. When Solomon sang to his lover, he didn't mention her good work habits:

> Your rounded thighs are like jewels, the work of a master hand. Your navel is a rounded bowl that never lacks mixed wine. Your belly is a heap of wheat, encircled with lilies. Your two breasts are like two fawns, twins of a gazelle. Your neck is like an ivory tower. Your eyes are pools in Heshbon, by the gate of Bathrabbim. Your nose is like a tower of Lebanon, overlooking Damascus. . . .

And when his lover described him, she didn't mention his IQ:

> His head is the finest gold; his locks are wavy, black as a raven. His eyes are like doves beside springs of water, bathed in milk, fitly set. His cheeks are like beds of spice,

yielding fragrance. His lips are lilies, distilling liquid myrrh. His arms are rounded gold, set with jewels. His body is ivory work, encrusted with sapphires. His legs are alabaster columns, set upon bases of gold. . . .

The Venus de Milo and Cleopatra, Cyrano de Bergerac and Snow White, Cinderella and the Phantom of the Opera and Miss America. The power of beauty—and the failings of ugliness—are reflected everywhere in the stories and artifacts of Western culture.

Appearance will affect us from our earliest hours ("What a pretty baby!") through death ("He looks so natural"). It will affect how we are treated as children, as students, as employees and professionals. Our relationships with relatives, friends, and complete strangers intimately involve matters of personal appearance. Appearance will affect how we mate and with whom.

A concern with personal appearance is natural. It is not a trivial concern, to be dismissed as vanity. To many people, a particular aspect of their appearance may be a decided handicap, no less debilitating than a missing hand or leg or eye.

More than a half-million Americans—mostly women, but an increasing proportion are men—go to board-certified plastic surgeons every year for aesthetic surgery. Thousands more go to surgeons certified in other specialties who have begun to do cosmetic surgery.

Most of these aesthetic-surgery patients are not rich, nor are they entertainers or potential beauty queens looking for a touch-up. Most are ordinary people, often quite thoughtful, who have become intensely aware of the penalties of poor personal appearance. They are willing to undergo financial hardships and, quite often, a substantial amount of pain to achieve an improvement in their appearance.

A nurse met the patient outside the elevator on the third floor, took her to a recovery room, showed her where she could lock up her street clothes and how to change into a hospital gown ("It ties in back, dear."). When the patient was ready, she walked with a nurse to a prep room in the operating suite.

In the prep room, she sat on the edge of a gurney—one of those wheeled beds that are always rushed down hallways in the hospital shows on TV—tipped her face up, and let the nurse wash it with pink antiseptic soap.

The scrubbing continued for several moments. It was gentle but thorough. When it was done, the nurse, a slender elderly lady with a kind face and gray hair, patted it dry with a sterile towel.

As the patient was being scrubbed, a Porsche 911 whipped down the still-dark street beside the hospital and disappeared around back. A few minutes later, its driver stepped through a back entrance and walked briskly down the dimmed hospital hallways. He was a sandy-haired, solidly built man—not fat, but sturdy, like a soccer player. A little taller than average, in his late thirties, he had pale blue eyes of the merciless shade supposedly possessed by the best of fighter pilots. He wore a conservative business suit and tie with a white shirt. He walked with the direct and confident air of a man at home in the very early hours, in a hospital.

His name is Bruce Cunningham, and he is a plastic and microsurgeon. He walked straight through to the operating suite and turned down a hallway to the prep room, still in his street clothes.

"There you are," he said to the patient, his face creasing with a broad smile. "How are you feeling?"

"Fine."

"Did you get enough sleep last night?"

"Some." The patient smiled tentatively.

"Well, you look great. I want to look at you for just a moment and talk about some things again. . . ."

Cunningham had already seen the patient twice. He had decided that she was a good candidate for a rhinoplasty, which would reduce the size and change the shape of her nose.

The determination of whether a person is a suitable candidate for plastic surgery is made on several points.

4

The feature to be corrected must depart from the norm in appearance. Further, the patient must be seeking the surgery for herself—the correction should not be sought because somebody else wants it. (Cunningham often sees teenaged girls whose affluent parents think a rhinoplasty is in order, while the girl herself doesn't seem too interested. He does not do those.) The patient must also have a rational attitude toward the operation, viewing it as the correction of a physical problem, without inflated expectations. In other words, a plastic surgeon can promise to straighten a nose, but can't promise a dramatic improvement in a person's love life.

The patient in this case fit all the criteria. Her nose, given contemporary standards of beauty, was notably oversized and sharply beaked. She considered it a serious problem of personal appearance and always had. She did not seem to be under pressure from her husband or members of her family to get the surgery. Her view of the situation seemed rational.

"It doesn't have to be beautiful. I just don't want it to be a big nose," she said. "If it's just an average nose, that would be fine. It doesn't have to be perfect."

Cunningham was a bit more ambitious than that. He wants a perfect nose every time.

There are places in some large metropolitan areas, especially on the West Coast, where a patient can essentially walk in for a rhinoplasty. In by ten, out by two. The operations are done in almost assembly-line fashion, and in a few of the places, all the noses come out looking roughly the same.

"There's a point where you stop being a surgeon and start being a mechanic," Cunningham said one day as he relaxed in his office at the University of Minnesota. "There are perfect noses for all the different kinds of faces, but there's not one perfect nose for all of them. If you see a signature nose, you're looking at a bad rhinoplasty."

Rhinoplasties, he said, are serious surgeries. Some surgeons, attempting to quiet fears of potential patients, have publicly suggested that rhinoplasties are no more complicated than routine tooth extractions. Cunningham said that opinion is terribly mistaken. The physiology and geometry of the nose are intensely complicated. A surgical error can do appalling damage.

"The patient is putting an incredible amount of trust in you. You are obligated to take it seriously. If you blow the operation out of negligence and get a bad result, then you've done just about the worst possible thing you could do to her. You took a person who came to you with a serious problem, and you made it worse. Everybody makes mistakes. But if you screw up because you're in a hurry to get to the next operation to make more money—that's indefensible," Cunningham said.

After Cunningham reexamined the patient, to make sure there had been no changes since the last office visit, he again cautioned her that the results might not be perfect—that problems do occur in surgery. The patient said she understood. He asked her if she had eaten, or taken any medication, including aspirin. She had not. Cunningham turned her over to the nurses and the anesthesiologist. The patient was rolled down to the operating room on the gurney, passively watching the ceiling tiles go by. The anesthesiologist explained to her about the sedatives that she would get intravenously, through a needle into her arm, and began hooking her up.

While the patient was taken to the operating room, Cunningham went to the men's locker room. He made a quick call to his secretary to confirm the day's schedule and then changed out of his street clothes and into his operating-room garments. When he was ready, he walked down to the operating room, where a nurse helped him into a sterile gown and gloves. The patient had been sedated, and by the time Cunningham had checked his tools and other surgical supplies, was sleeping soundly. Cunningham filled a syringe with local anesthetic and began the procedure.

The operation lasted about two hours. At one point, deep in

the work, Cunningham picked up a surgical chisel and said, "Now we're going to take that top right off." Ten minutes later, the beaked nose was a thing of the past.

At the completion of a rhinoplasty, the tissues of the nose have begun to swell with fluid, and some free blood has begun to seep under the skin below the eyes, giving the typical post-rhino black eyes. Nevertheless, the change in the patient was obvious. Her nose was finer, more delicate. The bridge was lower. Before the operation, her face might have been characterized as strong. Now she might be called beautiful.

Plastic surgery seems a magical process. While other kinds of surgeries attempt to heal the body, plastic surgeries have as much effect on the mind as on the body. And while plastic surgery may sometimes be denigrated as unimportant, as a sadomasochistic process performed by the greedy on the vain, the people who do the denigrating rarely need the surgery.

No one who has spoken to women who have had breast reductions or reconstructions, have had disfiguring noses rebuilt, have had ten years taken off their faces or double handfuls of extra skin taken off their stomachs, would claim that plastic surgery is without serious importance. The effect on many women is quite literally transfiguring.

And though in the end it is healing, plastic surgery is *surgery*. It involves a cutting of the mortal flesh. It can be both beautiful and brutal. It combines art with blood and pain. When a surgeon lifts a bundle of muscle, you can see the pale snaking lines of the nerves. Bones can be watched working around their joints, like living illustrations from a high school textbook. Translucent amber fat cells quiver like Jell-O molds just below the skin, and when burned with a surgical cautery, may send stinking smoke through an entire operating suite.

On good days, a facile surgeon will splice blood vessels as thin as Christmas-tree needles, with a dozen hand-tied square knots, each smaller than a period on this page. No normal human could do that; at its highest levels, the art of plastic surgery approaches the sublime.

On bad days, a surgeon will fight a losing battle to repair impossibly disfiguring burns, trying this, trying that, compromising, compromising. A bloody Rorschach spreads across his operating gown, gouts of nauseating smoke from a cautery stream into his face, weariness haunts his eyes, and he can never, ever quit. Surgery can be as ugly as an abattoir.

Cunningham never tires of it—not even of the routine surgeries, the facelifts or the rhinoplasties, which he refuses to call "nose jobs." Pressed on the matter, he reacts as an artist might: If you paint one good picture, that's no reason to quit doing it. You paint another. And another. Each is a challenge, and each is another chance at perfection. Surgery is his art; and nothing less.

In general, a plastic surgeon's work falls into two broad categories, aesthetic repair and functional repair.

Aesthetic repair attempts to improve appearance that might otherwise fall near the limits of the normal range. Rhinoplasties, facelifts, tummy tucks, breast enhancements, breast reductions, and suction lipectomies (the removal of localized deposits of fat) are examples.

Functional repair fixes human organs that don't work. The problem may be congenital—the patient was born with it—or may have been acquired in war, by accident, through other forms of violence, or from disease. Breast reconstructions after cancer surgery fall into this category. Burn repairs, which attempt to cover open wounds with new skin, are also in this category.

This book follows the work of a single experienced surgeon, Bruce Cunningham of the University of Minnesota. Through his work we see numerous cases taken from those two broad categories of plastic surgery, the aesthetic and the functional, including most of the major types of aesthetic surgeries.

Cunningham is also a skilled microsurgeon and does extremely complicated muscle transplants and replants; those operations will be discussed later.

And finally, we will look at an approach to an operation that is a sharp departure from all current plastic or microsurgical practice. Cunningham is a university surgeon and is expected to do research as well as the regular, established operations. It is a requirement he finds congenial: He has a taste for the experimental. For some time, he has been interested in the prospect of transplanting a hand from a brain-dead accident victim to a person who has lost one or both hands to accident or disease. He is now doing preliminary work toward that end, and we will take a brief look at that work.

All of this work—the aesthetic plastic surgery, the reconstructive plastic surgery, the hand transplant—has a common end. Stated quite simply, it is to make people work right or look better. To fix them. To bring them, or return them, from the shadows to a place where they can feel better about themselves—strengthened by aesthetic surgery.

Facelift

THE BEST time in a hospital is the early morning, when the nurses wake the patients and the orderlies begin to wheel them through the cool, quiet, half-lit corridors to the operating rooms. The first cases are on the operating tables at 7:00 A.M. or a few minutes later.

The morning medical staff is sharp with the start of another day, and there is a warm fraternity to the place. The business and office staffs, with their bureaucratic preoccupations, have not yet arrived. Nor are there people huffing through the corridors with complaints about bills, treatment, or any of the other problems that nag a major medical center.

It's a feeling of *just us medics, taking care of people.*

It's a feeling that disappears during banking hours, under a blizzard of memos, schedules, and hostile queries. The mood in the evening, when the business offices have closed, is even darker. There are no regularly scheduled surgeries at the end of the day. Those that take place involve emergencies: car accidents, explosions, burns, knifings, shootings, beatings, heart attacks, screaming patients and weeping families, operations done in a fog of blood on people soaked in alcohol and fighting the doctors every step of the way.

10

But the morning hours—the morning hours are the best. Locker-room conversations about baseball and surgery, *The Twins have lost fifty on the road, how in hell. . . . Opened up and looked at the joint and there was stuff coming out of there and I figured no way. . . . There were probably fifty or sixty people in there, and I'm saying to myself, wait a minute, nobody's smoking. . . .*

It's quiet. Made for medicine.

Cunningham lives at the distant western rim of the Twin Cities. He and his wife, who is also a plastic surgeon, wake in the dark, around 5:00 A.M. He works at four separate hospitals and two clinics, and most are a long drive from his home. It's seven o'clock by the time he arrives at that morning's first hospital. He stashes the car in the doctors' parking lot and heads for the locker room.

The nurses and surgical technicians are already working. The nurses prep patients who spent the night in the hospitals, greet and prep those who are arriving directly from their homes. The support services, equipment, and paperwork are checked. Surgical technicians begin preparing the operating rooms.

In the locker room—most hospital locker rooms are somewhat decrepit, like those in old downtown athletic clubs—Cunningham changes from his street clothes into a scrub suit. A typical scrub suit is a light, loose cotton shirt-and-pants combination, clean but nonsterile, stored in a large bin. Scrub suits are usually blue, green, or plum-colored. After dressing, Cunningham covers his hair with a paper hat, and his shoes with paper moccasins. Many surgeons wear running or gym shoes in the operating room, claiming that the soft soles are easier on the back. Cunningham does not; he stays with his street loafers. He also has minor back problems, but refuses to concede a connection.

Cunningham goes through this procedure every day; but this is a particular day, with a facelift first on the schedule.

When Cunningham walked into the operating room, the patient, a middle-aged woman, was lying faceup on the operating table. Her eyes were open, but she stared straight at the ceiling, unmoving. Her hands were at her sides. She was covered by a rough, off-white drape. She was relaxed, sleepy. Two circular ceiling-hung surgical lamps, each as big as an automobile tire, were focused on her face.

A surgical technician, dressed in a sterile blue operating gown, mask, and latex surgical gloves, sorted tools on two stainless-steel trays, with a light tink and clatter. A nurse in nonsterile surgical scrub suit sat on a stool, chatting with a resident (a surgeon in training) as she waited for orders. An anesthesiologist hovered behind the woman's head. When Cunningham looked at him, the anesthesiologist nodded and said he'd started a sedative.

Cunningham leaned over the table and looked directly into the woman's face.

"Feeling pretty good?" he asked.

"Pretty good," she said.

"We have to do a little drawing," Cunningham said. He showed her a surgical marking pen—similar to a dime-store marker, but filled with sterile ink and much more expensive—and she blinked at it.

Taking the blink as acknowledgment, Cunningham carefully drew a rough half-circle on the woman's face. The half-circle centered on a point in front of her ear and halfway down it. The rim of the circle touched the outside tip of her eyebrow, dipped into her cheek, slid past the corner of her mouth, dropped under her chin and onto her neck. It marked the limits of the skin that would be lifted away from underlying tissue.

The patient was in her late fifties, and, from a few feet away, strikingly attractive. Up close, her age was evident. Bags of excess skin on her eyelids gave her a hooded look. Her facial skin had a dry slackness to it, and crepey wrinkles crossed her cheeks. The skin and muscle under her chin had begun to sag.

Although the changes were slight, they were telltale. Five years earlier, a new acquaintance might have guessed her age as forty to forty-five, though at the time she was fifty-three. Now an observant new acquaintance would easily and accurately guess that her age was near sixty.

For some people, especially those concerned with appearance, that is a tragedy. As a practical matter, Americans consider age to be unattractive—and the bias is universal. It is held by both sexes and all ages and cultures and at all educational and economic levels. This patient, accustomed to the attention given a good-looking woman, would now be called a handsome elderly lady. She wasn't about to stand for it. Not yet. Her basic good looks and fine bone structure were made for a facelift. A skillful operation could take off a decade.

A facelift tightens loose skin and underlying tissues by pulling them back and up toward the ears. In addition to the basic lift, a complete facelift may include several additional procedures, any of which may be done independently, and often are.

The basic facelift is called a *rhytidectomy*. About 66,930 were performed in 1986 and 90 percent of them were done on women. They are one of the classic aesthetic surgeries, but are now surpassed in popularity by suction lipectomies (which reduce spot fat deposits), breast augmentations, and aesthetic surgeries on the nose and eyelids.

The other operations that may or may not be included in a full facelift are:

- The *blepharoplasty*, which is aesthetic surgery that cleans up sagging and tired-looking tissue above and below the eyes. As a separate operation, it is even more common than the full facelift, with some 84,690 now done by plastic surgeons annually.
- The *otoplasty*, which alters the shape or the set of the ears, and is often done on youngsters. Some 15,000 are now done by plastic surgeons annually.
- The *mentoplasty*, which improves the shape of the chin. More than 15,000 are done by plastic surgeons annually in the United States.
- The forehead lift, for which the American Society of Plastic and Reconstructive Surgeons lists no Greek-based name. About 16,000 are done by plastic surgeons annually.

Plastic surgeons also perform *dermabrasions* and *chemical peels*, which attempt to improve the quality of facial skin damaged by acne or other diseases, and *hair transplants*. The three operations are also done by dermatologists.

A rhinoplasty, or "nose job" (a label that most plastic surgeons despise; it sounds too much like plumbing), is not normally included as part of a facelift.

The face is the most critical operating arena for the plastic surgeon simply because it is visible. Small changes in complexion, cast, or shape may be the difference between the beautiful and the ugly. Cunningham brings a great deal of experience to the operating table, and because of the subtlety of the work, is meticulous in preparing the patient and drawing guidelines on the face.

With this particular patient, Cunningham took a full five minutes to lay down the guidelines. He gently manipulated the woman's skin as he worked, getting a feel for its quality. When he was satisfied, he leaned directly over her eyes again, so she could see him without straining.

"We're going to pin back your hair now, we're about to start," he told her, speaking slowly with careful enunciation. She nodded, and he picked up several steel clips from the tool tray and carefully pinned her hair away from her face. Halfway through the process, she closed her eyes, apparently dozing off. Cunningham glanced up at the anesthesiologist, who said, "She's okay."

When he finished pinning her hair, Cunningham picked up a syringe as long and thick as a big man's middle finger, with a long, flexible needle. The surgical technician held out a stainless-steel cup half full of liquid anesthetic, and he sucked up a syringeful.

"You're going to feel a little stick now," he said to the woman. She nodded sleepily. The needle was frighteningly large, but slipped easily through the skin—and then kept going in, and in, at a shallow angle to the surface. The woman showed no sign of pain or discomfort. Cunningham began injecting the anesthetic.

"Most people could never tell that a woman's had a facelift, if they didn't know about it in the first place," he said as he worked. He was hunched over the woman, his face only a few inches from hers. "I can tell sometimes. The tip-off isn't the face. The tip-off is that the woman looks younger than she acts. If a woman is getting close to sixty, and acts that way, but she looks like she's forty-five or fifty, I begin to think she might have had a facelift. Then, if you get close, sometimes you can see the scars down in front of the ears, though they're hard to spot. Most of the time the hair covers the scars anyway, and then you really can't tell."

Cunningham spent ten minutes squirting multiple small doses of anesthetic into the woman's face and the skin of her neck. Some of the puncture wounds bled a bit, leaving traces of blood on the woman's cheek.

"Are you warm enough?" he asked her as he put the needle down.

There was a long pause before the woman answered. When she did, her voice seemed to come from a distance, the words spoken with conscious effort: "Yes."

"Okay. We're going to wash you now."

Cunningham nodded to the resident, who would assist in the operation. The younger man leaned over the woman and said, "I'm going to wash your face now. I want you to close your eyes real tight. Okay?"

Pause. "Okay."

Cunningham left the room to scrub, and as the resident washed the woman's face, a nurse-anesthetist walked in. The anesthesiologist, who induced the anesthesia, is a doctor. A nurse-anesthetist is a registered nurse with lengthy advanced work in the specialty of anesthesia. After a briefing on the progress of the work, she took over for the anesthesiologist, who left for another operation. The anesthetist checked her monitoring equipment and asked the patient if she felt comfortable.

Pause. "Fine."

"You're not lying on a wrinkle or anything?"

Pause. "No."

Anesthetist: "Would you like some music?"

Pause. "Sure."

Anesthetist: "What would you like?"

Pause. "Classical. Something . . . light."

"Oh, good," said the resident. "We won't have to listen to rock."

Pause. "Not Mahler."

"Oh, yeah, I wouldn't want to do a facelift to Mahler. Or Wagner," said the resident as he massaged her face with pink antiseptic soap.

Pause. "Oh, God. No."

The woman had a small, relaxed smile on her face. As the resident continued to scrub her, the nurse-anesthetist tried to tune an old bread-loaf-sized brown plastic radio. She cranked through several stations whose music was either egregiously offensive or whose reception was markedly unsteady, and finally landed on an easy-listening station. Radios don't seem to work well in operating rooms.

Operating rooms are like windowless bunkers, isolated from outside activities. The walls feel thick and protective. Architecturally, operating rooms resemble incredibly clean public bathrooms, all beige tile and terrazzo. Glass-fronted, stainless-steel cabinets full of drugs and common surgical equipment line the walls. Everything looks easily and often washed.

The operating table is the focus of the room. Patient-monitoring gear is stacked on carts around one end of it. Stainless-steel equipment tables and tool trays are set to one side, where they can easily be reached by the surgical tech.

Before an operation, all the beige tile and stainless steel serve as a kind of psychologically cool anticolor scheme. During an operation, however, the dominant color in the room is an intense, vibrating blue. It's the color of the sterile gowns—worn over the scrub suits—and the hats, masks, and shoe-covers worn by the surgeons and technicians, and of the drapes and towels that cover the tables, the patient, and anything else that will come in contact with sterile personnel or equipment.

Operating rooms are kept warm so that patient temperature can be more easily controlled. They are well lit, with auxiliary overhead lights providing blazing illumination for the surgical field.

The overall feeling is one of control. Everything has a place, everything has a technique. Radios, however, don't work very well.

While the nurse-anesthetist looked for a decent radio station and the resident washed the patient's face, Cunningham was giving his hands a thorough scrubbing at the stainless-steel scrub sink just outside the operating room doors. He would wear sterile gloves while operating, but gloves have been known to tear, and to be nicked by scalpels, so there's nothing halfhearted about the scrubbing. Each finger is worked over, the nails are scrubbed with specially sealed, one-use brushes, and the arms are washed to the elbows.

Isolated from the task of surgery, Cunningham's hands do not look especially remarkable. But they are: Another surgeon, watching him operate, would say that Cunningham has "good hands."

His "good hands" look ordinary enough. Square, well tended, and somewhat soft, they might be the hands of any businessman. Their peculiar abilities become apparent only in the operating theater. They can make the finest, smallest movements; to watch them tie a gnat-sized knot is to smile at the virtuosity. They can be absolutely still. They are hands that could thread a needle twenty times out of twenty, fifty out of fifty.

In fact, his "good hands" are not just hands. He has the ability to conceptualize an operation, to plan it in his mind, move by move, and even to outline it on a restaurant napkin days before it is to take place, with a textbook clarity. The mind makes the hands better—and Cunningham has been training himself for his work since he was a child.

"I have a composition I wrote when I was in fifth or sixth grade, saying I wanted to go into medicine so I could help people," Cunningham said one day. "I've been pretty consistent about wanting to be a doctor. When I was in high school, I got a job as a scrub tech in a hospital. It was different then—they didn't have the training programs for scrub techs like they do now. You just went through an apprenticeship. The nurses told us what to do, and the surgeons trained us in.

"I'd go down to the pathology lab at night and use the operating microscope to dissect specimens that the lab didn't need anymore. . . .

"For most of the time I was an undergraduate in college, I thought I wanted to be a psychiatrist. I think that was just the normal rebellion against your father. [Cunningham's is also a surgeon.] Surgeons and psychiatrists are supposedly at opposite ends of the medical spectrum. You know, the surgeon is the dumb macho guy with a low forehead who does things but doesn't know anything, and the psychiatrist is this foppish wimp who knows everything but can't do anything. That's all total bullshit, of course. . . .

"So I read a lot of Freud and the post-Freudians, and it was fascinating, but ultimately it became clear that I'd be completely frustrated as a psychiatrist. Everything is too nebulous, you never know exactly where you are, what the variables are. I'm results-oriented, I want immediate gratification, I like to do something and see how it comes out."

When Cunningham finished scrubbing, he shook the loose water from his hands and held them upright, away from his body, in the familiar TV-surgeon position, and bumped hip-first back through the swinging operating-room doors. He arrived just as the nurse-anesthetist finished fine-tuning the easy-listening radio station. The surgeon cocked his head at the music and frowned over his mask.

"What's this? Could we find some music that won't terrorize our brains?" He moved up next to the operating table, his hands still hung out in the air, and looked down at the patient.

"Do you like jazz?" he asked.

Pause. "No."

"Okay," Cunningham said. He turned to the anesthetist. "Look around ninety-two. You'll find some decent classical there."

As the anesthetist went back to tuning the radio, the surgical technician helped Cunningham into his sterile gown and gloves. The resident finished washing the patient's face, rinsed the soap off with sterile saline solution, and wiped it dry with sterile towels. When he finished, Cunningham bent over the patient again, took her face in his gloved hands, and gently turned it.

"Numb," she said.

"What's that?" asked Cunningham.

"My face. It's numb."

"Yeah, it looks like it's starting to get there," Cunningham said. Cunningham turned to an observer: "You see how her skin has turned white? There's [the drug] epinephrine in the anesthetic. It constricts the blood vessels and limits the blood loss. Sometimes we'll be doing a job under general anesthetic, and we'll use the local [anesthetic] anyway just to get the epinephrine effect."

The circulating nurse had left the room when Cunningham came in, and now returned pushing a chair.

"Just what the doctor ordered," she said when she came in. She pushed it up behind him and, with help from the surgical tech, covered it with a sterile blue drape. Cunningham sat down and picked up the surgical marker.

The original markings had faded when the resident scrubbed the woman's face, and Cunningham quickly sketched them back in. He showed the resident where the incisions would go and explained why he would lift some areas of skin and not others.

"We want to go under both sides of her jaw," he said, pointing with the marker. "If she were heavy, we might want to go all the way under, so everything is loose. If you get somebody who is really obese, you might want to make another incision along this line [he drew a line under the woman's chin] and either suck out some fat or carve it out."

When he was sure the resident understood the sequence, Cunningham picked up a small scalpel and made the first incision. It was a shallow vertical cut down the front of the ear. Because of the epinephrine, there was almost no blood.

The first cut in an operation is always interesting. It reaffirms what most people don't wish to think about, but which is crystal clear in surgery: what lies below the human skin is meat. It looks like meat and has the raw smell of meat.

After making the single short incision, Cunningham picked up a pair of forceps—they look like big tweezers. Working with the scalpel in one hand and the forceps in the other, he carefully freed the edge of the facial skin from the underlying tissue. When he had a flap an inch or so wide, he discarded the forceps and scalpel, picked up a large needle, and sewed six-inch lengths of thread into the top and bottom of the flap of skin. The threads would be used as handles so the resident could pull up on the facial skin as Cunningham worked beneath it.

As Cunningham worked into the face, he occasionally cut through an active blood vessel, and blood would trickle into the wound. Using an instrument called a cautery, which looks like a big ballpoint pen or a small soldering iron, the bleeding vessels were sealed with electric sparks. Each spark sent a small puff of smoke into the air, and the room was quickly suffused with the odor of burning blood. It's exactly the same pungent organic burning smell of a tooth drilled a bit too vigorously.

With the resident tugging on the two thread-ties, pulling the skin away from the face, Cunningham began to free more skin from the underlying tissue. After he was in a short distance, he traded the scalpel for a small pair of scissors. There was a rapid sequence: tiny, tiny snips, then a quick zap with a cautery, a puff of smoke, and more snips.

"See those little black dots [on the underside of the skin]? Those are the bottom of the hair follicles," Cunningham noted as he worked beneath a sideburn near the top of the ear. The dots looked like facial blackheads. "When you're under the hairline like this, you have to be careful to cut deep enough that you don't injure the hair follicles. If you do, you'll leave her with an area of baldness. On the other hand, you don't want to cut so deep that you risk injuring the nerve that goes to her forehead."

Nerve damage is one of the most drastic risks of facelifts. It is not common, but it can happen. If critical nerves are badly damaged, the affected muscles may be left paralyzed and will eventually wither.

Because of that small but real risk, the separation of skin from underlying tissue is slow and meticulous work, about what you'd expect from a two-thousand-dollar haircut. The skin is thin, though not particularly delicate. Watching the scissors work below it is like watching the surface of a taut bed sheet while your feet move around beneath it.

When the skin was loosened out to the limits of the half-circle drawn on the patient's face—to the corner of the eye, the corner of the mouth, and under the chin—Cunningham stitched two more lengths of thread into the rim of the ear. The resident used them as handles to pull the ear forward, and Cunningham made a second incision behind it. Working through the relatively short cut, he undermined the skin on the side of the woman's neck.

As he worked he hit a bleeder and sealed it with a quick zap of the cautery. The woman flinched.

"Is that painful back there?"

Nothing.

"Did you feel that?"

Pause. "Just a little, just then."

Cunningham looked over at the surgical technician: "Some anesthetic, please?" The surgical tech handed him the syringe and held the cup of anesthetic so he could suck some up. Then to the woman: "Now this is the anesthetic going in."

He made several more injections in the neck and waited a moment for the anesthetic to take effect. When he resumed, the woman showed no awareness of the work. He finished with the neck a few moments later and went back to the cheek. Using scissors again, he began loosening the thin layer of fat that clings to the facial muscles and lies just below the skin.

"Look right there," he said, lifting the loosened fat layer with the tip of the scissors. "You see those white lines? Those are the facial nerves. Cut those, and you have big problems." The nerves looked like pieces of extremely fine, well-cooked spaghetti against the deep purple cheek muscle.

When the layer of facial fat had been freed, the preliminary work on the right side of the face was complete. The skin and fat now lay loosely over the cheek, rather like a wet cloth.

The next stage, the actual tightening of the facial layers, began immediately. Cunningham, gripping the fat layer with his fingers, tugged it up toward the ear and looked at it for a moment, fitting it. When he was satisfied, he quickly sutured it to the cheek muscles in front of the ear. A band of excess fat, perhaps an eighth of an inch thick, extended over the ear itself, and was neatly trimmed away.

Areas of the woman's face that had been slack were suddenly and visibly firmer.

"Show me your teeth," Cunningham said to the woman.

After a moment's delay, she pulled back her lips in a grimace.

"Good," he said. He looked up at the resident. "We want to make sure we haven't somehow put pressure on those facial nerves, and you can get an idea about the level of sedation by the way she responds."

Leaving the skin loose on the right side of the face, he rolled the patient's face to the other side. Picking up the marker, he drew another set of guidelines. The anesthetist leaned over the patient and said, "We're going to do some more injecting, so we're going to make you sleepy again. Do you feel more sleepy?"

Long pause. "No," she said weakly.

She sounded much sleepier than when she was asked to show her teeth. The anesthetist nodded to Cunningham, who began another series of injections with the long needle. A few moments later, he made the first incision on the left side of the woman's face. The operation was going well, and Cunningham and the resident exchanged small talk as they worked.

"You decide yet what you're going to do?" Cunningham asked

at one point, referring to the resident's imminent decision on a specialty.

"Medicine, I guess," said the resident.

"Jeez, I don't know about that," said Cunningham, wiggling his eyebrows. "If you can do good surgery, why go into a field where you have to think?"

The resident wiggled his own eyebrows in a wordless acknowledgment of the mild jab.

Because the doctors, nurses, and technicians in an operating room are robed and masked, and their hands are occupied, they can't use the normal facial and body cues common to all conversation. They compensate with their eyes and their eyebrows, reflecting anger, boredom, contempt, agreement with a cast of the eyes.

Cunningham commented on this. "The hierarchy in a surgical situation is so fixed that you're limited in the ways you can speak and the tone of the voice you can use, and you're forced to dissemble in the way you release your anger or anxieties," he said. "If a surgeon gets tense and barks at a nurse, she can't turn around and say 'You goddamn asshole' without disrupting the whole flow of the place. But she can say 'Yes, sir' and roll her eyes up so far in her head that everybody in the place knows she's saying, 'Sit on this, Jack.' "

Cunningham freed the skin on the left side of the woman's face, then the fat layer, and repeated the procedures done on the right side. When he finished, he rolled her head back to the right and began the final stage, the suturing of the incisions.

He was now a little more than two hours into the operation and approaching the critical stage. He must pull the skin tight, to get the requested firmness, but he had to take care not to put too much pressure along the line of the incision.

A primary cause of heavy scarring is pressure or tension on a wound. If the wound is arranged so that natural muscle movement will put stress across the incision, the scarring can be serious—and almost any scarring will defeat the purpose of a facelift.

"When you pull the skin up [toward the ear], you naturally get some tension. You have to find a place to put it, so you suspend the whole works from two stitches, one right at the top of the ear, and one right behind it," Cunningham explained. He pulled the facial skin tight across the right side of the patient's face and put in the two stitches.

"This way, the pressure that might otherwise go on the developing scar will go on the stitches instead. If we put those two stitches up in the hairline above the ear, and behind the ear, you can hide the scars where nobody will ever see them. Neat, huh?"

With the two suspension stitches in place, he carefully lined up the edges of the wound.

"Stapler."

The surgical tech handed him a stapler not markedly different from an office stapler, and he began stapling the edges of the wound that lay within the hairline. Staples are used only within the hairline because they leave behind tiny dotlike scars that might be visible on the open face.

When the staples were in, Cunningham and the resident closed the remainder of the incision with a long running stitch, using tiny needles and fine nylon thread. The stitch, which would be on the open face, had almost no pressure on it. Its scar would be as fine as a baby's hair.

With the incision at the front of the ear neatly closed, Cunningham placed a drain in the wound behind the ear. The drain— a flat plastic tube that trailed out of the wound and down the back of the patient's neck—would siphon out any fluid that collected in the wound. An accumulation of fluid could put pressure on the wound and intensify scarring. With the drain in place and working, the procedure was repeated on the other side of the woman's face.

Though the patient had not yet left the operating table, she already looked better. The trauma of surgery causes some immediate swelling and distortion of facial tissues, but it was evident that her face was tauter and more angular than it had been before the operation. She looked younger.

"The next part sounds worst to most people, when you talk

about it, but it's really not bad at all," Cunningham said. "Most people are just very sensitive about their eyes."

As the woman had grown older, her eyelids had stretched and become looser, giving her a heavy-lidded look that people unconsciously associate with age.

Cunningham, using the marker again, drew two baselines across the patient's eyelids. Then, with a small pair of tweezers, he pinched the excess skin together.

"That's about as much as we should take. You can see that we can take it without putting any undue pressure on the lid."

He indicated the limits of the cut with the marker and then repeated the sequence on the other lid. When he was done, he had two small football-shaped lozenges marked on her eyelids.

"I'm going to do some injecting now," he said to the woman. "You're going to feel a little pain in your eyes." She said nothing, and Cunningham began injecting anesthetic into the skin of her eyelids with a very fine needle.

When he was satisfied that the drug was working properly, he picked up a small scalpel and tiny hooklike retractors. Making very light, fine incisions, he cut loose the first scrap of eyelid skin.

"If there's a fat problem, you can go into the compartment behind the lid and take out some of the fat," he told the resident as they worked. "That's not a problem here."

With the first scrap of skin freed, the wound was covered with a gauze pad soaked in saline solution, to keep it damp. The two doctors moved to the second lid.

"If you do this right, the suture scar will be right on the fold line, and totally invisible," Cunningham said. The second scrap came free. The two wounds were quickly and neatly sewn up with fine thread.

The operation had been under way for a little more than three and a half hours, and the surgical crew began to get restless as the end came in sight. The nurses talked about lunch, and Cunningham, a movie enthusiast, talked about seeing *Kiss of the Spider Woman*.

"I couldn't stand that," said the surgical tech, a young woman.

25

"I turned it off as soon as the two guys went to bed together."

"I guess that got to some people," Cunningham said amiably. He turned to the resident: "She [the patient] is going to stay overnight in a hotel and come back in tomorrow to have those drains taken out."

"Okay."

"Let me tell you about William Hurt," he said, turning back to the surgical tech, "I thought he was just excellent. What an unbelievable role . . ."

After the final stitch went into the eyelid, Cunningham bandaged the woman's face with an over-the-head, under-the-chin technique, like the bandages put on toothaches in old newspaper cartoons.

"The idea is to hold everything in place and let it heal," Cunningham said. The woman, though she looked sleepy, was now almost fully awake and listening.

"We're all done," Cunningham said, bending over her. "Everything went fine. I'll see you tomorrow."

"Okay . . . thanks." She still sounded distant, but was rapidly waking up. Cunningham stripped off his operating gown and gloves and headed for the locker room.

Cunningham enjoys facelifts, just as he enjoys rhinoplasties. They are comfortable operations with a degree of art to them, and they produce gratifying responses from the patients.

But to Cunningham, the facelifts are routine, and one blends into another. A month after an operation, he has to look at his records to remember the work on a particular patient, unless there was something distinctly odd about the patient or the procedure.

It is exactly the opposite with patients. They remember not only Cunningham, but every circumstance of the operation. For the patients, the operation is a once-in-a-lifetime matter, accompanied by deep anticipation, some fear, and a little pain.

In early 1987, Cunningham did facelifts on three women his secretary called "the three amigos." The women were longtime friends. They had their preliminary examinations on the same day, and all three decided to go ahead with the operations. Later, they provided mutual support as each went through the facelift.

Two of the three agreed to be interviewed about their operations. The two are sisters, Anne and Beth, ages sixty-seven and sixty-five. The sisters were enthusiastic when discussing their facelifts. They were interviewed about three months after Anne's operation, and a month after Beth's.

Anne had fully recovered; Beth was experiencing some residual numbness, but it was fading.

"We'd been talking about getting facelifts for years," said Anne. "I checked with another doctor at University Hospitals, and he recommended Dr. Cunningham. So we set up an appointment."

The sisters had somewhat different problems.

Anne, a widow, had severe wrinkling on her cheeks and some loose skin beneath her neck. Beth had some wrinkling, but not to the extent that Anne did. On the other hand, Beth had a large mass of loose skin on her neck that had always made her feel self-conscious. The problems had developed when the women were in their late forties and grew increasingly severe during their fifties.

"The only thing I really regret about the operation is that I didn't have it while [my husband] was alive," Anne said.

Both had stories concerning their appearance.

Anne told of a time when her young grandson came to the house on Halloween wearing a costume and black makeup.

"I gave him a big hug, like I always did, and he said, 'Oh, Grandma, you got black stuff all over your face.' So I wiped it off and said, 'There, did I get it all?' And he said, 'Yes, most of it—it's only in the cracks now.' "

Anne remembered the comment for seventeen years.

Beth and Anne related a story about a mutual friend who was visiting Anne, but had not seen either sister for several years. Anne showed him a picture of Beth, and he said, "Gee, she's gotten fat."

"I said, 'She's not fat, she's only one hundred twenty pounds.' He was looking at that loose skin under her neck and thought it was fat," Anne said.

"I had it pretty bad," Beth admitted. "I called it a turkey neck, but it wasn't very funny when you had it. I looked in the mirror and I thought, Gee, is this really me?"

Something, they decided individually, had to be done. The obvious thing was a facelift.

"I wasn't scared, exactly. I guess the only thing that made me nervous was that I saw an operation on TV, you know, where you see the blood and everything. That made me a little nervous, but I don't think I was too bad," said Beth.

Both operations were done with sedation and local anesthetics, but not full anesthesia. Both women could remember parts of the procedures.

"I remember him talking about the scissors when he was doing my eye . . . and then I could feel the clipping. Not exactly pain, but I could feel it, so I told him. I said, 'I can feel that now,' and he said, 'Okay, we'll give you another shot,' " said Beth. "Later on, I remember hearing the little staple gun going, and I thought, My God, is that a staple gun? It sounds like they're putting down carpeting."

Neither felt much pain after surgery. Beth said she was uncomfortable for a short time when the sedation began to wear off, "but it wasn't anything serious." Cunningham had prescribed pain pills for her, but the discomfort was so transitory that she took only a few of them during the course of recovery.

Anne suffered some nausea during the recovery, but didn't feel much pain at all. Cunningham also gave her pain pills, but she didn't take any.

Anne had had several operations over the course of her life, and said that the pain from the facelift had been comparatively minor. Beth had never had surgery before, but did suffer migraine headaches. She said the pain of the operation was much less severe than a migraine.

"The operation was nothing compared to a migraine. I'd rather have ten operations like this facelift than have one migraine," she said.

Anne said that she had not had her upper eyelids tightened as Beth had, and was planning to go back for that work. "So that's about how much it hurt me. I've already decided to do another one," she said.

The two sisters said they had radically different amounts of bruising. Anne had extensive black-and blue marks, while Beth had practically none at all—"One bruise about the size of a dime."

"I went shopping five days after the surgery," Anne related. "My daughter is in the beauty business and got me some makeup, some cover-up, and that took care of the problem."

Beth was out shopping three days after the operation.

"The only thing that really bothered me about the operation was the staples," Beth said. "They're kind of uncomfortable. I couldn't wear my glasses because they were pushing back there. Then you start to think that they might be loosening up, but you push them a little bit and they seem to stick. I had him take a couple out so I could use my glasses. They were a little bit uncomfortable," said Beth.

She added: "When you ask what hurt the most, I can tell you. I can say, 'This did' or 'That did.' Or the staples. But none of it hurt very much.

"The worst thing in the first couple of days was looking in the mirror and seeing all those stitches. I was thinking, Oh, my God, what did I let him do to me? But then the stitches came out, and everything was fine."

Anne said that it was interesting to be the first of the three to be operated on, "because then the other girls would call me up after their operations and say, 'This happened, now what?' And I could say, 'Oh, that happened to me, too, but don't worry, it'll go away.' Like Beth says she still feels a little numb on her chin. So did I. But it went away."

Both women said the operation made them feel better about their appearance, and that their friends had remarked on how good they looked. Friends who had not been told about the operation remarked on their appearance, but did not ask if they'd had facelifts.

"I don't really care if people know—but it was interesting that people who we didn't tell, didn't guess," Anne said.

She expects her daughters to have the same procedure.

"We waited too long, I think. We should have had it done years ago. Dr. Cunningham said the usual time is in the early and middle fifties. I wish I had had mine then," she said.

Both women, now in their middle sixties, are quite attractive. Seen in a store or on the sidewalk, a passerby might guess their ages as between fifty and fifty-five.

Snapshot: The Team

Most Americans like teams and teamwork. We like to be on the team, part of the team. We are taught to work as teams from the first days in a sandlot, in Boy Scouts and Girl Scouts, in the military, and in business.

We expect a team to be something more than the sum of its parts. A true team has emotional and spiritual ties—team spirit. The members are assumed to be familiar with one another, to compensate for individual weaknesses, to rely on individual strengths. Team members are not required to be friends, but are expected to have strong bonds.

The people who gather in an operating suite to perform surgery are called *surgical teams*. In truth, they are something more and something less than ordinary teams.

Surgical teams don't have the personal ties of true teams. Rarely will the same doctors and nurses work with one another two days in a row. Too many things intervene—days off, vacations, scheduling changes, shift rotations.

The differences in social and professional status also work against a true team feeling. Doctors are usually well-paid independent contractors and bear virtually all responsibility for the outcome of an operation. Nurses and technicians are employees.

Yet, despite the barriers, there *is* a team spirit in an operating room. It grows from professionalism. A high level of performance is expected and rather routinely delivered. There are obvious and well-publicized exceptions to the rule, but they are rarities.

A surgical team consists of a minimum of four people: a surgeon, an anesthesiologist (or nurse-anesthetist), a surgical technician, and a circulating nurse. A resident, who is a doctor undergoing advanced training, is frequently on hand, as are medical students. Specialists commonly found in operating rooms include radiologists (doctors specializing in interpretation of X rays and electronic images) and X-ray technicians, mechanics, scientists, photographers, orderlies, and laboratory technicians of various ranks.

The surgeon is the team captain. He runs the operating room. What he says, goes. ("If he says spit in the wound, you spit in the wound," said a nurse. "Of course, when the operation's over, you turn him in.") When everything goes right, the surgeon gets the glory. If it turns sour, he bears the responsibility. Aside from his formal position, the surgeon sets the mood in an operating room. When he is serious and intent, the others are serious and intent. When he loosens up, they loosen up. When he talks, they talk; when he doesn't, they usually don't.

Frequently there is more than one surgeon in the operating room. Complex operations may be done by groups of surgeons working together. In many cases, the group consists of a lead surgeon, who is in overall charge of the operation, and any number of additional specialist surgeons. The specialists are not lower-ranking surgeons. They are in charge of their part of the operation.

In other cases, one surgeon will lead an operation, and others will simply assist. The assisting surgeons perform work that must be completed simultaneously with the main effort. In that case, the assisting surgeons *are* subordinate to the lead surgeon. But they are not always subordinate—in another operation, they may be the leaders, and others the assistants.

Surgery is a conservative art. Surgeons work by consensus. If there is not a consensus on surgical treatment of a particular patient, attending surgeons will go to almost any lengths to reach one. If a consensus can't be reached, dissenting surgeons may withdraw. The rule is fairly simple: the midway point in an operation is not a good place to argue basic procedure.

Surgeons are routinely assisted in their work by hospital residents, who are physicians in training. Residents have their M.D. degrees and are serving an apprenticeship in whatever specialty attracts them. Depending on the level of residency (the number of years they've served) they may assist in very elementary ways or do a complete operation by themselves under the watchful eye of the staff surgeon.

Surgeons tend to have substantial egos. Part of it involves social status: working surgeons are the survivors of a rigorous academic and practical testing, which lesser lights have failed. They do challenging, intellectual, humanitarian work, to virtually universal approbation. They are their own bosses, earn large amounts of money, drive expensive cars, and eat in the best restaurants. They are small gods in the operating rooms.

Given the circumstances, ego is inevitable. It's also necessary. It takes an exceptionally strong personality to pick up a knife and inflict a desperate wound on another human being, with the full confidence that the wound can be repaired. And it's not just a matter of a surgeon nerving himself up for an occasional operation. Laymen, familiar with operating suites mainly through television, are often astonished at how many operations a real surgeon will do. General surgeons may do two or three a day; specialists even more. In trauma centers, one lead surgeon, with assistance from residents, will sometimes handle two operations simultaneously, involving radically different injuries to completely different body structures.

And while each television surgery is an event involving heavy tension, deep breathing, tight jaws, and sweaty foreheads, life for most surgeons is much more routine. They are known to hum, sing, and even whistle while they work. The very best surgeons are most alive with scalpels in their hands.

Cunningham is heavily involved in surgery. He operates almost every weekday, and sometimes does two, three, or four surgeries on the same day. His bread-and-butter is the standard repertoire of the aesthetic surgeon: facelifts, tummy tucks, breast enhancements and reductions, and rhinoplasties. His services are in demand. His rhinoplasties are routinely booked two and three months ahead. A few surgeries are booked ahead eight, nine, and ten months.

In addition to the aesthetic surgery, he does the routine non-aesthetic work expected of every plastic surgeon: skin grafts and skin expansions, scar revisions, the removal of moles and skin cancers, and breast reconstructions.

His most esoteric work involves microsurgery on tiny physical structures like nerves and blood vessels. He can take a muscle from one part of the body and move it to another, where it's needed, tying in the blood vessels at the new site. He does this in the hot light of a microscope, using needles no bigger than eyelashes and thread so thin it can barely be seen with the naked eye.

He likes it.

"There's no end to surgery. You can always do it better, no matter how well you do it, and there's always the possibility that something unexpected is waiting. You just don't know for sure until you make that first cut, and after you do that, there's no backing away—you've got to do something. When you're working, you can get in so deep, it's like there's nothing else but you and the work.

"Sometimes when I'm doing a free flap [muscle transplant], I get to a point where I don't even know what else is going on; they'd have to tell me if the OR caught fire," he said.

The "other" medical doctor always around an operating room is the anesthesiologist. He induces and controls anesthesia of the patient and generally monitors the patient's life signs during the operation. He is usually assisted by a nurse-anesthetist. In routine operations, anesthesia is usually induced and lifted under the supervision of an anesthesiologist, while the nurse-anesthetist monitors the patient during the operation. There is *always* somebody at the anesthesia post during an operation.

A surgical technician—also called a scrub tech—directly assists the surgeon, passing instruments and other equipment, or occasionally holding a retractor in place. The technician is garbed entirely in sterile clothing, just as the surgeon is. Usually the tech is the first person into the operating room and sets it up for the operation. In the past, most surgical techs have been nurses. Increasingly frequently, the tech is not a nurse but a graduate of a separate year-long training course at a vocational-technical school. In the latter case, the tech is not qualified to make the patient-care decisions handled by registered nurses.

Circulating nurses—all operations have at least one, and there are sometimes several—provide the necessary medical supplies for the operation and perform other backup work. During the course of an operation, a surgeon may need a whole range of supplies: drugs, blood, bags of saline solution, towels, sponges, additional instruments, even chairs. He may also need informational support, like laboratory results or chart information. Information is simply spoken across the room. Supplies are a more complicated proposition.

Within the operating room, there are two distinct groups of people: the sterile and the nonsterile.

The sterile people, the surgeons and surgical technicians, may not touch anything nonsterile. If a nonsterile thing is touched, the clothing that made contact is considered contaminated and is changed.

The nonsterile people, on the other hand, may not touch anything sterile. If they do, the now nonsterile covering is either replaced or covered with another sterile robe. In some operating rooms, nonsterile people are not permitted even to walk between two sterile areas.

This sharp separation creates a barrier, but it is frequently necessary to move medical supplies across it without contamination. The technique for doing so is straightforward, but to the layman may at first seem odd.

Asked for sterile gauze pads, a circulating nurse picks up the specially designed package containing the pads. The package is usually transparent plastic, so she can see what's inside. It is shaped something like the hamburger cartons that Big Macs and

Quarter Pounders are delivered in. Gripping the package on opposite sides, the nurse pulls it apart as though she were opening a clamshell. The nurse never touches the gauze pads or the inside of the package.

The sterile-gloved surgical tech carefully reaches into the open package and takes out the sterile gauze. She never touches the outside of the package or allows the gauze to touch it. The barrier is crossed, and the sterile remains sterile.

All supplies are handled the same way, from gauze pads to needles and thread to electronic instruments. Even the surgeon's robes come in special packages, nonsterile on the outside, sterile on the inside.

Working together, the surgical tech and the circulating nurse move supplies across the sterile barrier without breaking it.

Like soldiers, medical people are intensely aware of rank. In the operating room, the surgeon is at the top, followed by any other doctor, including the anesthesiologist and residents.

Nurses and degree-holding technicians are next. Surgical techs, unless they're nurses themselves, rank below the registered nurses, but above the practical nurses. Practical nurses are a step above the orderlies and other housekeeping personnel. Special duties and special competency may alter these rankings, but not by much, and not very often.

The status differences are reinforced by dress codes, some formal, some informal.

In many hospitals, only fully qualified staff doctors wear knee-length white coats. Hospital residents, one rung down the ladder, also wear full-length coats, but colored rather than white. Medical students, a rather large rung down, wear white coats like the staff doctors, but shorter, just hip-length.

Under these coverings, doctors almost always wear suits and neckties, even if they are female. (There is a young macho subgroup of doctors, of both sexes, who tend to dress more informally, apparently under the influence of "M*A*S*H" and "St.

Elsewhere." The rebellion doesn't amount to much, however, and usually dies out by their mid-thirties.)

Nurses usually wear uniforms with name-and-rank tags. If they are specialists (nurse-practitioner, nurse-anesthetist), the tag says so. If they have Ph.D., M.A., or B.S. degrees, the tag says that, too. If they are working in an office that requires business dress, they often wear stethoscopes around their necks to distinguish themselves from nonmedical office workers.

Hospital administrators tend to dress like doctors, but don't get to wear the long white coats. Volunteer workers may wear special dress that testifies to their status (gray ladies, candy-stripers).

Orderlies, who exist at the lowest level of the hospital pecking order, wear long knee-length white coats just like the doctors. The major distinguishing feature is that the orderlies' coats have stains on them—orderlies carry around pans of unsavory things that are sometimes spilled. In addition to the stains, orderlies are also distinguished by the lack of a suit and necktie, which are *de rigueur* for the doctors themselves.

A simple rule of thumb: if you meet an orderly with a necktie, you've encountered a man who just doesn't give a damn.

For the most part, rank differences, accepted as necessary to efficiency, go unchallenged and unspoken. But things are not always that peaceful. Surgeons are known to demonstrate their rank in the operating room with temper tantrums, during which they throw instruments and curse assistants. The abuse is never returned within the operating room, or even challenged. In that place, at that time, too much is at stake. Later, outside the room, the situation may be different—support personnel have both formal and informal ways of striking back at abusive surgeons.

When a surgeon has a temper tantrum and becomes unduly abusive, he will often apologize on the spot. Most doctors want a good working relationship with support people. It makes life easier. Operating staffs tend to be forgiving, knowing the pressure under which the surgeon works.

"I've blown up once or twice, usually out of frustration or anger with myself. I never really had much of a problem that way, though," said Cunningham, who has a reputation of being a fairly mellow surgeon. "The stories of surgeons going berserk are classics, and there are surgeons who do it all the time. I remember when I was a scrub tech working in surgery and how I felt when somebody blew up at me. I felt horrible if I had done something stupid, and so indignant and angry when it wasn't something I was responsible for, but there wasn't a thing I could say or do. You feel powerless. I think that memory is a restraining factor whenever I start getting a little tense."

With some surgeons, the abuse becomes chronic. On rare occasion, an unrepentant surgeon has been forced by hospital executives to apologize for misbehavior or face the loss of staff privileges.

There are other, less formal penalties for abusive behavior.

Nurses generally determine a surgeon's social acceptability around a hospital. A mean-spirited cutter is quickly designated a jerk.

Once a surgeon is designated a jerk (and the designation is quickly picked up by other hospital personnel, including other doctors) everybody is a bit wary of him.

To be designated as a jerk is to find a certain coldness in life. An operating room can be quite a friendly, informal, and even cheerful place; it can also be quite formal, unpleasant, and dreary. Most doctors find life on the jerk list to be unpleasant. Others have been known to maintain their status for years, and apparently take some pride in it.

Those who do make a conscious effort to improve their status will eventually get off the list, and may later get a certain gentle joshing about their former attitude. One thing is quite clear: only the nurses can get a reformed jerk off the list.

Appearance

THE FACE is the vial of the soul.

The Plains Indians knew it. Crazy Horse, the great mystic warrior, refused to sit for a photographic portrait: he feared his spirit would be trapped in the image.

The Romans knew it. Roman actors wore masks—interchangeable faces—to reflect moral roles in their plays. Our English word *person* is derived from *persona*, the Latin word for those masks. Just as a Roman actor's mask portrayed wealth or poverty, stress or serenity, age or youth, pleasure or pain, attraction or repulsion, so does a person's face.

The face discloses the smallest, most fleeting emotion and the broadest, most intimate excitements. It is not by accident that erotic scenes in good movies focus as much on the face as on the body. Nor is it an accident that conservative Moslem nations require women to go masked: the face, it is believed, is such an intimate part of a woman's personality that no man should look on it but her husband.

The face has always played a critical role in art. How many people would not recognize the Mona Lisa in an instant? How many would not recognize the farmer and his daughter in Grant

Wood's *American Gothic*? Artists from El Greco to Larry Rivers have distorted faces, and particularly the eyes, because of the powerful effect such distortions have on the viewer.

A startling drawing produced by the nineteenth-century American artist Thomas Eakins portrays a nude and grossly obese woman. Her face is wrapped with a black cloth.

The black wrapping was not a comment on the misproportioned body: it was an effort to preserve the model's privacy in Victorian times. But the mask robs the model of her individuality, of her history. The viewer is not allowed to search her face for the signs of moral corruption or intellectual debasement that might provide a convenient explanation for the decrepit body. Nor does Eakins present the woman as an allegory, as an illustration of the wages of sin.

The Eakins drawing says, "Here she is. Look at her. A woman served an ugliness she does not necessarily deserve." Ugliness, the drawing argues, does not always have meaning. Sometimes, it simply *is*.

The powerful reactions elicited by the Eakins drawing suggest that we intuitively recognize ugliness as a curse of the first magnitude. We instinctively know that it may be absolutely unrelated to an individual's virtues or vices. By extension, the reverse argument is made for beauty: that it is a great benefit—Aristotle considered beauty a gift of the gods—completely unrelated to personal virtue. We even joke about the injustice of it: "Men seldom make passes at girls who wear glasses." "Blondes have more fun."

We acknowledge both the curse and the gift with our everyday actions. We turn away from the ugly ("Jimmy, don't stare at the poor man!") and toward the beautiful. Every magazine rack in the nation cries out with the power of the beautiful face.

With feelings about appearance so powerful and so universal, it might be thought natural that a person would attempt to improve his or her appearance. And it *is* thought natural, to a point. Hairdressing is natural, makeup is natural, flattering clothing is natural.

For most of recent history, surgery was considered unnatural. The only excuse was severe disfiguration, like a missing nose or a missing lip. Purely optional aesthetic surgery was thought by many people to be the epitome of vanity—and even to carry a little purple fringe of masochism. Go through all that pain and expense for a neater nose? She must have something wrong with her.

A sizable number of professional psychologists and psychotherapists once agreed with that sentiment. They argued that aesthetic surgery was a symptom of neurosis, or worse. A person who wished to change his or her appearance, they felt, must have a shaky self-identity or a faulty relationship with reality. The cure for that was in therapy, not in surgery. Surgery simply pandered to the neurosis, rather than attending to the root of the problem.

So the young girl has a nose like the best Idaho baked potato? Help her adjust to reality. Reducing the spud to a neat, symmetrical French fry is too easy an answer.

That was the argument in many of the learned journals. To an extent, it still exists (and in certain cases, is clearly applicable). The argument didn't mean much to the American public. While the therapists debated and wrote papers, Americans, saturated with televised examples of the power of beauty, ignored them and flocked to the plastic surgeons.

The American Society of Plastic and Reconstructive Surgeons reports that its members did 590,580 aesthetic surgeries in 1986, up sharply from 477,700 just two years before.

There were also 1,850,310 reconstructive surgeries of various kinds, ranging from aesthetic-functional operations like elaborate breast reconstructions to straightforward functional work on cuts, dog bites, skin cancers, and burns.

The opinions of the psychologists are changing, too. There is now a good deal of scientific evidence that appearance is critical to success or failure in life—and that an attempt to change a bad appearance might represent distinctly rational behavior. Good appearance—to a point—is a positive aid in a person's relationships with others, the scientists now concede. Bad appearance is a distinct, if not insuperable, barrier to success.

(Ironically, significant research shows that therapists and counselors who once suspected that plastic surgery was evidence of neurosis are no more immune to the effects of beauty and ugliness than anyone else. Attractive patients tend to get better treatment and more personal attention from therapists and tend to make faster recoveries.)

One clever study of attractiveness was done by a researcher who sent questionnaires to county public health administrators, asking for guidance in her career choice. The researcher, posing as an undergraduate student, asked the administrators to recommend a graduate college in public health administration; asked what her chances were of getting into such a school; and asked for an estimate of her chances of getting a good job in public health administration after she graduated.

The questions were accompanied by a résumé. Some résumés included a photo of an unattractively obese woman, others a photo of a woman of normal weight (actually, the same woman; in the "fat" photo, her clothes had been padded). A third set of résumés had no photo attached, nor did it state a weight.

The "good photo" or "no photo" résumés got replies from 57 to 65 percent of the administrators. The "fat photo" résumés got answers less than 25 percent of the time. Most of the administrators who replied to the "fat photo" résumé suggested that schools were hard to get into and jobs scarce. The other résumés got much more encouraging replies.

Studies by other psychologists and sociologists have confirmed this finding again and again. Even professional personnel managers discriminate for the attractive—and often they do it consciously.

Research shows that candidates for managerial posts must look the part of the job, as well as have the requisite abilities, if they wish to be hired. Some scientists thought it possible that personnel managers would hire people who most resembled themselves—not notably worse, but not notably better, either. That proposition was quickly disproven: even unattractive personnel managers favored the attractive.

A standard college text on abnormal psychology cites research that indicates college men talk differently on the telephone to women they believe to be attractive than to women they believe to be unattractive. The women picked up their attitude (over the phone!) and reacted accordingly. Neutral observers, asked to listen to the conversations, could identify which women the male callers believed to be unattractive.

Ellen Berscheid, editor of the journal *Contemporary Psychology* and one of the leading authorities on the psychological effects of appearance, has a straightforward answer to why good appearance is so important.

"It's wired in," she said, meaning that it's part of our basic biological makeup.

She cited an elaborate study done with infants using two screens suspended above the babies' cribs. The screens were controlled by the way the infants turned their heads. If the baby's head turned one way, one screen would show an attractive adult. If the baby's head was turned the other, the adult was unattractive. The babies showed a significant preference for the attractive adult, Berscheid said.

"So it's wired into our brain. One possible reason is that a good appearance is related to health and physical fitness. The choice to associate with those kinds of people could be a survival choice, a matter of propagation of the species. There really hasn't been much work done in that particular area, not what there needs to be."

Berscheid is chary of generalizing from specific studies: too many generalizations are later found to be wrong, based on unperceived prejudices.

But she says flatly, "One of the most robust, unquestionable findings that we have is that attractiveness provides positive social advantages to those who possess it."

If beauty is so important then, exactly what is it? Who's pretty, and who's not? If all this research has been done, there must be some formula.

There is not.

Beauty is like pornography. You know it when you see it, but getting an objective description is another matter. One problem with finding a definition is that beauty does not necessarily involve a specific set of physical features. A beautiful person may be blond or raven-haired, round or oval-faced, tall or slight. So may an unattractive person. A woman may be attractive or unattractive depending on how she feels, or how she feels about herself, and that can change from time to time, and even hour to hour.

Women who have had beauty "make-overs" at salons may go from drab ugly ducklings to beautiful swans in a day or so, with the results shaped artificially by proper clothing, hairstyles, and makeup. Lose the clothing, hairstyle, and makeup, and it's back to duckling.

Psychologists have generally given up trying to define beauty and ugliness. Instead, they use an ad hoc definition—that beautiful, average, or ugly people are those whom a representative sample of the population say are beautiful, average, or ugly. They find remarkable agreement in those calls.

Berscheid warns that anyone thinking about plastic surgery as a way to improve personal appearance is setting foot on a slippery path. "I couldn't recommend that anyone have, or not have, plastic surgery without actually getting to know the person and each individual situation. Everything is so difficult," she said.

It is perfectly possible, she said, to imagine a person who believes that a rhinoplasty would help improve his appearance and that the improved appearance would lead to a better social life. So that person has the nose job, and his social life does, indeed, improve—not because the old nose was ugly, but because his attitude toward his social life has changed. His personal self-esteem may have risen, he may be more confident and outgoing.

It is also possible to imagine the reverse case, where a person believes that a rhinoplasty will improve his social life, has the operation, and waits—and nothing happens. The problem was not his nose, but personality traits that other people found unattractive. And he hasn't changed those.

Finally, it's quite possible to imagine a person with a very unusual nose, who is otherwise happy with his life and appearance. He gets the nose changed without expecting or getting any big change in life. The rhinoplasty represents an aesthetic decision, a purchase to make the recipient happy, just as someone else might buy a Picasso.

"It's impossible to tell without looking at the individual," Berscheid said. "There are some cases of disfigurement, where you just say, 'Do it,' but most cases are a lot more complicated than that."

She also suggested that a decision on whether to have plastic surgery might involve a shrewd assessment of personal circumstances. If a person has a somewhat awkward nose, for instance, a decision about a rhinoplasty might depend on his job.

"If the job involves a lot of onetime social interactions, like sales work, then you might want to have it changed. When you're in those onetime situations, attractiveness can be very important. I think it becomes less important as your onetime social contacts become fewer. If you have a job where you work with just a few people, who come to know you well, I think the personality becomes more important and the physical traits less so."

Beauty is not necessarily an unalloyed gift, Berscheid added.

"One time I was asked to give a speech to a gathering of dentists and oral surgeons and so on, and these guys were stunned by what I was telling them [about the importance of attractiveness].

"Now, I hate to travel, and I was feeling sick that day. I had a cold and a fever and I just wanted to get back to my hotel room, but on my way out after the speech I ran into this cluster of men. They nabbed me, and they said, 'We've been talking about our kids. We want to know what you think we should do if we have kids who are physically unattractive. Should they get surgery and all that, to try to make them attractive? Is it that important?'

"And I said, just off the top of my head because I was tired and sick, 'If they're smart, don't do anything; if they're dumb, try to make them attractive.' And I took off. Later I was lying on my bed and I thought, My God, what did I just do to those guys?"

She said, though, that she is tempted to defend that offhand standard, more because of personal feelings than because of research. Beauty, she explained, can be a distraction. It's a gift, but it has its price. If an adolescent girl is beautiful, and has lots of attention and a heavy social schedule, she may not develop other talents she might have. Those other talents, Berscheid thinks, will be more important in the long run.

"Because we all get old, and age is unattractive. A person who is just beautiful is going to lose that, and all the other talents she might have had will be lost, too, if they're not developed.

"What I'm saying, and I really don't have any research to back this up, is that beauty provides a path of least resistance. It's very seductive. A lot of people are happy to take it. If he or she has no other talents, then that may be the only choice. If there are other talents, those should be developed. They'll last. That's why I said what I did to those oral surgeons."

Beauty is so emphasized in American society that Berscheid fears for the future of pretty women.

"Men are traditionally pushed toward success in some special area, so even if they're handsome, that's not enough. With women, it's different. If you're beautiful, it can be enough, at least to survive on. If you fall into that, the other things never get developed," she said.

But attractiveness, good appearance, is important?

"Oh, yes. No question."

If appearance is so important, why shouldn't everybody simply go for it—go for the best appearance they could possibly have, and damn the pain and discomfort?

Because it's not realistic.

"Surgery is expensive," Berscheid said, "and there are other priorities. I don't think anyone would argue that a person with limited resources should go for a small improvement in appearance, at great cost, while they neglect something like education."

So cost-benefit considerations are important, too. Surgery is not cheap.

Surgical costs vary widely from one hospital to another, from one region to the next, from one country to another, and from surgeon to surgeon. Generally, however, the least expensive types of surgery will cost as much as a modest used car. For the typical prices of the more expensive surgeries, you could buy a rather nice new car. In certain cases, plastic surgeons may become "stars"—often by doing creditable work on entertainment personalities. The fees charged by these surgeons range from the extraordinary to the outrageous—we are now in Mercedes-Benz territory.

Almost no aesthetic plastic surgery is covered by insurance, although in some cases, as with breast reduction operations, that may be changing.

Because appearance is so important, men and women have always sought ways to improve their looks. Egyptian doctors were attempting surgical repairs of the nose before Aristotle started philosophizing about beauty. They apparently had some success with their procedures—their rhinoplasties are recorded in hieroglyphics on papyrus scrolls.

Ceramic artists in India three thousand years ago were constructing false noses for people who had lost theirs to combat or disease. An Indian doctor who lived seven hundred years before Christ described both nose and earlobe reconstructions. Chinese doctors were repairing harelips fifteen hundred years ago. Pre-Norman Celts and other early Europeans also fixed harelips.

There are reliable reports of complex plastic surgeries done in Italy in the 1400s and 1500s. The next two hundred years, however, saw a general decline in the sophistication of plastic surgery, as erroneous notions and theories about wound care took root in the European medical establishment. One tragic error involved the belief that tissue could be transplanted from a donor—like a slave—to a recipient, to repair disfiguring wounds. Modern medicine knows this to be impossible because of immune reactions. But the repeated transplant attempts of the seventeenth and eighteenth centuries, with the consequent failures, cast a shadow on the whole field of aesthetic surgery.

By the beginning of the nineteenth century, progress had resumed. British physicians were discussing the reconstruction of noses by Indian surgeons, operations widely reported in reputable medical journals. These Indian surgeons, using a sophisticated "flap" method, borrowed living skin from the patient's forehead for use in reconstructing the nose. The technique is still used today. (Indians were particularly interested in rhinoplasties because the loss of a nose in their society carried a social stigma. Amputation of the nose was punishment for a variety of crimes, including adultery and theft. It was also a punishment occasionally visited upon the losers of a battle.)

The renewed interest in plastic surgery can partially be attributed to the rise of the mass army. As late as the mid-eighteenth century, armies were still relatively small by modern standards. A major battle might involve a few thousand men on each side and seldom lasted more than a day or two.

After the revolutionary era of the eighteenth century, armies were numbered in the tens and hundreds of thousands, and battles had become relentless and seemingly unending campaigns. Soldiers were exposed to violence for days and weeks on end.

The face is in particular danger in battle. The reason is simple and brutal: if you can't see and breathe, you can't fight. During moments of highest danger, the face is usually turned toward the threat. As a result, it is frequently wounded. And unlike wounds to other parts of the body, even superficial wounds to the face can be socially and psychologically crippling. Facial scarring may be even more devastating than the loss of a penis or the testicles, because those losses at least can be concealed.

Before the present century, the alternatives for men disfigured in combat were distressing. The deformity and functional loss could be accepted by the victim, but acceptance usually meant a limited, reclusive life away from society. Surgery—without anesthesia—was another option, but results were often limited to functional repair. Aesthetic improvement was a much more difficult and unlikely proposition. A final option for these men was death.

In the introduction to *Reconstructive Plastic Surgery*, a standard work in the field, author John Marquis Converse quoted the renowned sixteenth-century surgeon André Pare on the aftermath of a battle:

Having arrived in town, I entered a stable and there I found four soldiers who were dead and three who were leaning against the wall, their faces completely disfigured and they could not see nor could they hear or speak and their clothes were still smoking from the gun powder that had burnt them. As I was looking at them in pity, an old soldier approached me and asked me if there was any way by which I could cure them: I answered that there was no way. Suddenly he approached each one of them and cut his throat, gently and without anger. Seeing this cruel action I told him that he was a bad man to have done this. He answered that he prayed God that if he should be so afflicted there would be someone who would render him the same service rather than allow him to languish in misery.

As armies became more modern and developed weapons such as shrapnel, the problems of disfigurement grew worse. Trench warfare protected the bodies of defenders quite well, but necessarily left the faces, especially the eyes, exposed at critical moments. Shrapnel often creates great tearing wounds without killing.

During World War I, the casualty lists were appalling. Thousands of men suffered disfiguring injuries, so many that the French victims formed a lobbying group called Les Gueules Cassées, or "The Broken Faces," to seek aid from government facilities.

The results of modern warfare could stir even the most hardened of correspondents.

Ernest Hemingway, in *A Moveable Feast*, his memoir of Paris after World War I:

> There were other people too who lived in the quarter and came to the Lilas [café], and some of them wore the Croix de Guerre ribbons in their lapels and others also had the yellow and green of the Médaille Militaire, and I watched how well they were overcoming the handicap of the loss of limbs, and saw the quality of their artificial eyes and the degree of skill with which their faces had been reconstructed. There was always an almost iridescent shiny cast about the considerably reconstructed face, rather like that of a well packed ski run, and we respected these clients. . . .

The decades between World War I and World War II saw sweeping improvements in anesthetic, antiseptic, and surgical techniques. Skin grafts became practical. World War II, the first really worldwide war fought with modern machinery, also presented doctors with a wider range of common, survivable wounds that would require the services of plastic surgeons—everything from frostbite to severe burns to various kinds of tropical skin rot.

The wars of the twentieth century gave plastic surgeons great scope for research and plenty of practical work. Military physicians set up the first regular plastic surgical units to provide specialized care for victims of disfiguring wounds. Dental surgeons became involved in reconstructive efforts, doing much work in the area of aesthetic prosthetic devices.

The work done in the military hospitals was carried by the physicians back into civilian life, where it was applied to victims of more routine accidents—automobile collisions, industrial explosions, home mishaps.

At the beginning of the twentieth century, plastic-surgery techniques were rudimentary. By the last quarter century, all that had changed.

Techniques of local anesthesia are now sophisticated enough to handle operations previously done only under general anesthesia. And general anesthesia has become much safer. Surgical techniques have been refined. Plastic surgery is no longer limited to the attempted repair of grotesque deformities. Purely elective surgery, for relatively minor defects, is not only possible, but even popular.

Although aesthetic surgery is becoming increasingly common, cultural differences still affect its general popularity. In the United States, plastic surgery is relatively most popular in states with the largest urban populations, and especially those that have traditionally been entertainment centers—New York, Los Angeles, Miami, Las Vegas. It is relatively less popular in the South and Midwest.

The growth in plastic surgery is not just a phenomenon of the media-saturated United States. It is becoming increasingly accepted all through the non-Communist world. Anywhere there is an established middle class, able to afford the luxury of non-lifesaving surgery, there are top-class plastic surgeons to do the work.

The leading edge of plastic surgery research has traditionally been in Britain, France, Germany, and the United States. The fastest-spreading operation in the history of plastic surgery, for example, is the suction lipectomy, and it was developed in the 1970s in France. Leading journals of plastic surgery routinely feature reports on work done in Mexico and South America, the Middle East and Japan and Singapore, along with those from western Europe and the United States.

Plastic surgeons also tend to be an international group. Many non-U.S. surgeons received their training in the United States, and many American surgeons have gone abroad for training seminars and to observe new methods of plastic surgery.

In the 1980s, plastic and reconstructive surgery became the most rapidly growing of all surgical fields.

The growth is accelerating.

Snapshot: Tools

The first person who shows up for work in an operating room is the surgical technician. The tech checks her assignments for the day and then, with the help of a circulating nurse, assembles the tools needed by the surgeons she will assist.

To begin, either the tech or a circulating nurse brings in the needed tool kits. The kits are stainless-steel pans about the size of roasting pans. The tools inside the pans have been washed after their last use and then sterilized inside the pan. The pan has been closed since the sterilization process.

If the tech brings in the tool pans, she removes the lids and sets them aside. She is careful not to touch the sterile tools inside the pans. Then she leaves the operating room and scrubs thoroughly with antiseptic soap at a special scrub sink. Once scrubbed, she puts on a sterile gown and gloves with the help of a circulating nurse.

When she is gowned, with the help of a circulating nurse she spreads sterile blue paper sheets (called *drapes*) across the tool tables, the operating table, and any other surface that needs to be sterile. Taking care not to touch the unsterile exterior of the tool kits, she removes the tools one by one and arranges them on the sterile drape, as though she were setting a dinner table.

Most of the tools are stainless steel; some are nickel-plated brass. There are cups and bowls and syringes, but mostly there are glittering silver-colored hand-held instruments for cutting and pulling and snipping. They have the cold, efficient, nasty look of weapons. The most striking thing about them is their primitive quality.

"We don't use anything that would surprise a carpenter," Cunningham said one day as he was rummaging through a rhinoplasty kit, with its special tools for nose surgery. "Knives, saws, files, chisels, it's all in there."

The difference between carpentry tools and a surgeon's instruments is not so much in kind as in quality and delicacy. The surgeon's instruments are the *very best* in knives, saws, files, chisels, pliers, and hammers.

There is some high technology, too. You'll hardly find a university surgery department without a few lasers tucked away somewhere, and everybody has an operating microscope or two. But by and large, most high-tech gear is used in diagnosis or the monitoring of a patient. The actual work of surgery is done with knives and their toolbox kin.

A scalpel is generally about the length of a pencil and made of stainless steel. It feels cold and solid and precise in the hand: not too light, not too heavy. A scalpel drawn across the skin will cut of its own weight, but not deeply. Modern scalpels have replaceable blades, like X-acto knives (which they much resemble). A surgeon may use several scalpels during an operation, but more commonly will just use one or two.

The bigger scalpels, used in general surgery for heavy work, are gripped like you'd grip a paring knife. Smaller blades, used in plastic and microsurgery, are gripped like pencils.

Surgeons occasionally use knives ten inches long and more, with square ends, resembling huge straight razors. They are used to strip away large areas of damaged muscle and skin, as must be done with burn victims.

Most surgeons do not say "Scalpel" when they want a scalpel; they say "Knife." How they work with the knife depends on the job at hand and, to some extent, on the surgeon's personality. Some work slowly and intently, some go at it with an almost gay panache. Cunningham blends his knife work into the rest of the operative routine. If you don't watch him closely, you can miss critical incisions—it's "syringe . . . knife . . . retractors" in a smooth, low-key process that downplays the pivotal nature of the first incisions.

Most scalpels are delicate. Chisels, used to shave bone, are not. Most of them look like common Sears, Roebuck cold chisels, though the cutting edge is much sharper, like the tip on a sculptor's wood chisel. Chisels are sharpened before each use on an ordinary whetstone and are hit with a stainless-steel hammer the size of a small ballpeen. Surgeons also use rasps to remove bone. They are slender steel instruments that may resemble a bicycle spoke with one roughened end.

Saws are used to cut bone. Some are hand-driven and some are electric. Some are made of flexible threads of steel, which are looped under a bone then whipped back and forth by hand until the bone is severed (similar to saws sold to naïve campers as "survival saws").

Surgeons use a wide variety of pliers, tweezers, clamps, and clips. Tweezers and pliers are used to manipulate tissue and other instruments (like needles). Hemostats are clamps that look like manicuring scissors and are used for everything from clamping blood vessels to fastening a surgical drape in place. Hemostats can be quite large, as big as a pair of sewing scissors. Other clamps are tiny and may look like delicate brass pen points.

Drills, like saws, come in both electric and hand-driven models to suit the job. Some look disconcertingly old-fashioned, the brace-and-bit kind that disappeared from most wood shops in the '50s and now are most often found at garage sales.

A cautery is an electrical instrument that looks like a delicate soldering iron and is one of the most-used instruments in surgery. It seals severed blood vessels by burning them shut with an electric spark. It may also be used like a scalpel, to cut through some kinds of connective tissue.

Because of its job, a cautery is an unpleasant instrument. Each use produces puffs of smoke from burned blood and tissue, and the burning smell is sharp, coppery, and repugnant.

The most common and benign-looking instruments in an operating room are the retractors. Retractors are used to pull tissue out of the way of the knife or other instruments. Some are tiny hooks, no bigger than an *s* in one of these words. Attached to stainless-steel handles, they look like the world's most expensive nut-picks. Other retractors may be as large as a man's hand, with tongs as big as fingers.

One special kind of retractor is called a fiber-optic. The end is lit (through glass fibers that carry light into the tip of the retractor) so that a surgeon can work under a large mass of tissue, like a breast, and still be able to see clearly.

The use of retractors produces one of the more interesting surprises in an operating room. Retraction often is—often must be—extremely vigorous. That is, if a surgeon is working under a breast with a scalpel, scissors, or a cautery, the breast tissue must be held firmly and unfailingly out of the way. It would not do for the resident suddenly to let a large mass of breast tissue slip off a retractor and smack down on top of a scalpel.

For that reason, when tissue is retracted, it is held with a firmness that may seem damaging—bruising. And, in fact, bruising is not uncommon in some types of surgery, especially deep abdominal surgery on obese people where large masses of fat must be tugged out of the way.

Retraction bruising is uncommon in plastic surgery, although some retractions may leave a layman observer feeling a bit queasy. When incisions are made inside a nose, for example, the nostril is pulled open with a small hook. What was a narrow, tidy opening at the bottom of the nose is suddenly stretched to the size of a dime. The patient feels nothing, but the act may bring sympathetic tears to the eyes of lay observers.

Some of the most intricate work in surgery is done with needle and thread, putting back together what the scalpel has cut apart. The sewing needles used in surgery are short, curved, and quite rigid, and range in length from three quarters of an inch to an inch and a half long or longer. They are not threaded like sewing needles, through an eye. Instead, the thread comes preattached to the tail of the needle.

The smallest needles are so delicate that if they are dropped, it is most difficult to find them again. (But they must be found, to be sure that they are not floating around in the wound. To find them, the nurses use a magnet to sweep across the floor of the operating room.) These needles, most often used in micro-surgery, are no bigger than an eyelash and use thread thinner than spider webbing. The thread can't be seen by the naked eye except under lights, and then only from certain angles.

Needles are manipulated with the fingers or with needle hold-ers, also called needle drivers or needle rams. The needle holders look something like a pair of manicure scissors. And though they have finger loops like scissors, only rookie surgeons use them that way. Most experienced surgeons hold the blades of the needle driver between their thumb and index finger, with the finger loops pressed into the palm.

The scissors used in surgery would be comfortable in a well-stocked sewing basket and vary in size from that of manicure scissors to out-and-out shears.

There are, of course, hypodermic needles around operating tables, universally called syringes. They range from small, dis-posable, pencil-thin instruments with tiny sharp glittering needles, to large pumplike devices with barrels as big around as a thumb, mounting needles two inches long.

There are also actual pumps—vacuum-cleaner–like devices used to suck blood and other fluids, and sometimes fat or smoke, from the operating field. Nurses at one hospital call them "slurps."

Operating rooms come with a variety of bottles, pans, and buckets to hold used sponges, bandages, and pieces of flesh re-moved from the patient. If the patient is catheterized, the plastic catheter tube will lead over the side of the table to a urine receptacle on the floor. And there is usually a garbage pail around, lined with a plastic bag.

One of the more complicated pieces of operating-room equip-ment is the table itself. It's narrow and long, and has arms that fold out from the sides to form a crucifix shape. The patient may lie either face up or face down; in the latter position, special pillows may be used under his chest and hips to keep him firmly in place. The face-down position may also require special sup-ports to make sure breathing tubes are not crimped or thrust against the back of the patient's throat.

57

At the head of the table is the anesthesia equipment, the most sophisticated electronic gear in the operating room. Included are heart, respiration, and temperature monitors, respiration aids, and racks for intravenous anesthetic and saline feeds.

The people who inhabit an operating room are all specially garbed in nonsterile masks, paper hats, shoe covers, and scrub suits. Those members of the staff who work under sterile conditions—the surgeons and the surgical technicians—are wrapped in long sterile gowns and wear thin, sterile latex gloves.

This gear is used by virtually all surgeons. Plastic and microsurgeons also use some special equipment.

One such instrument is the massive operating microscope, used to illuminate delicate structures like veins, arteries, nerves, and tendons. The scopes are mounted on wheeled stands and are pushed into place over the table when the surgeon is ready for them. Like the surgeon, an operating microscope is wrapped in a sterile gown or drape before it is wheeled into place. Most scopes have two eyepieces so both the surgeon and an assistant can look at the same operating field from opposite sides of the table.

Another optical aid is the loupe, which is essentially a set of matched magnifying glasses built into a pair of spectacles. The barrel-shaped loupes, usually three-quarters of an inch across and an inch or so long, protrude through the lenses of the spectacles. Seen the first time, they rather comically bring to mind the bug-eyes of the old cartoon crows Heckle and Jeckle.

Plastic surgeons in the past few years have been more and more frequently using devices called expanders, which are buried under the skin (and sometimes under the muscles) to expand overlying tissue.

In a patient with a severe burn of limited size, for example, expanders may be buried on either side of the burn scar to stretch the good skin. After it is stretched enough, a process that may take several weeks, the expanders are removed. The scar tissue is then cut away, and the extra skin produced by stretching is extended over the burned area. When this is done skillfully, a major scar can be reduced to a hairline.

Plastic surgeons also use a variety of pads and pieces of plastic to reshape breasts, chins, and other bodily parts.

The most unpleasant of the tools routinely used by plastic surgeons is called a dermatome. It's unpleasant both because of the noise it makes, and because of what it does.

The dermatome looks a little like an electric sander, but it acts more like a sod cutter—and it's used to harvest skin for skin grafts, just as sod is lifted in long strips from a field. It makes an unpleasant buzzing sound (reminiscent of the sound of a dentist's drill) as it cuts and leaves behind a strip of raw, bleeding skin. The harvested skin, which comes out the back of the machine, looks like a piece of thin, flexible, flesh-colored tape.

Many times, and especially in burn cases where large amounts of skin may be needed, the skin is placed on another tool called a mesher, which simply meshes the skin—turns it into a net. This allows the skin to be stretched to cover more area. The skin itself will grow back into the mesh holes, providing a solid cover, although the resultant scarring will give the healed surface a webbed appearance.

In addition to all the standard gear, Cunningham has been known to toss entire operating suites to find a radio and, once he has procured one, to devote substantial energy to finding just the right station.

"One time, you never heard of radios in operating rooms," said one nurse. "Now a surgeon with a radio is conservative. Some of these guys bring in these big ghetto-blasters with three hours of Mozart tapes, and they can't operate unless the tape is right. Jeez."

The Nose

"A GOOD rhinoplasty is a complicated operation," Cunningham said one day as he sprawled comfortably on a couch in his University office. "I don't know how many I've done. Thousands. I love to do them. I've studied it so long, I feel I can be [here he struggled for the right word] expressive. You can be *expressive* doing this work."

The nose is the most noticeable and striking facial feature, after the eyes. As an organ substantially unsupported by bone, totally exposed to the elements, and peculiarly affected by disease and heredity, it can stray far from what's generally accepted as normal. It can be sharp like a can opener or fat like a potato. It can be turned up and flattened, leaving the owner "pug-ugly." It can be twisted or pushed to one side, giving the eyes an untrustworthy look. The nose alone can make a man ugly, leave a woman shunned.

"I had a young girl in here not long ago, a teenager. I'd say she had one of the biggest noses I've ever seen. We really helped her out—not a Hollywood nose, but a real good nose. Even with the bruising and everything, you got that kind of reaction from her [when the bandages were removed] that makes the job worth it," Cunningham said lazily.

A Hollywood nose?

"Yeah, you know, one of these nice little cute angular noses with a scooped-out bridge and a flip on the end? Let me tell you, I get parents in here sometimes with their daughters, and the kid's nose isn't too bad, and the kid doesn't seem too interested in the operation. You talk to them for a while and you start to get the idea: they want a Hollywood nose.

"Like, this is not really a nose at all. It's an advertisement. It says, see, I have the money and the moxie to go downtown and get a nose job.

"The problem is, the girl has to live with the nose. Someday she'll be thirty-five years old. Maybe she's a lawyer moving toward a position of authority, and right in the middle of her face will be this cute little phony flip. She'll look like a teenager with real bad wrinkles instead of a mature human being," Cunningham said.

When Cunningham gets rolling with a story his eyebrows jump up and down and he moves his fingers and hands as though he is modeling in clay. He is a nonfat man who can look merry when he wishes, and he often does when he's story-telling.

"So I knew this woman years ago. She was small and thin and pretty, with this cute little Hollywood nose in the middle of her face. A real munchkin. She was left with no real strategy in dealing with the world, except to be cute.

"She had a lot of brains and she was in a field where she had to take authority. But how can you do that when everybody treats you like a kewpie doll? It's a problem. And I'll tell you, it's a lot easier to get a Hollywood nose than it is to fix one later," he said.

The rule followed by ethical surgeons, Cunningham said, is simple enough: the ideal rhinoplasty should never look like a rhinoplasty. The patient should look as though she were born with an attractive nose well fit to her face.

This is all very tricky water, especially when dealing with a patient who wants her nose to hint of surgery.

If patients do not get the success they expect, however, they tend to complain, loudly, and sometimes in the courts: "He said my nose would be beautiful, but Norma Jean still won't go out with me, so my nose must not be beautiful." He doesn't want to hear the argument that Norma Jean still thinks he's a jerk. (If the personality problem is a defensive reaction based on a genuinely unfortunate proboscis, however, a rhinoplasty may actually work wonders, and help a jerk take a long step toward becoming a nice guy.)

With most patients, their reason for seeking a rhinoplasty is evident the moment they walk into Cunningham's office. They know what they want, why they want it, and don't expect to be Cinderella. What they get is what they expect. A decent, nice-looking nose.

Rhinoplasties are the classic plastic surgery, with a history that can be traced back more than three thousand years. *Rhinoplasty* means "nose-forming" and derives from the same Greek root word as *rhinoceros*, which means "horny-nosed."

Rhinoplasties are the most common cosmetic surgeries performed on males, with more than 20,000 done on male patients in 1986. They are popular with women, too. Some 62,000 rhinoplasties were performed on female patients in 1986, trailing only suction lipectomies (removal of pockets of diet-resistant fat) and blepharoplasties (the removal of loose skin around the eyes) in the number done.

At one time, not long ago, some psychiatric theorists suggested that a rhinoplasty might be harmful to the male psyche.

"Men have two major midline organs," Cunningham said with a small smile. "The idea was that men identified one with the other. So if you put a guy under the knife and whittled down his nose—well, this might have some deleterious effects on the other organ. That has not proved to be the case. Fortunately."

Aesthetic problems involving the nose come in many forms. The most common requests are for overall size reduction, for removal of a hump, for a narrower nose, for a reduction in nostril size, or for a straighter nose. Frequently, a patient with a bulbous nose will have almost no bridge, and the surgeon will build one while simultaneously cutting down the top. Occasionally, especially with male athletes, a badly broken and flattened nose will be built up.

In the most common operation, to reduce nose size, the cartilage that supports the wings of the nose will be narrowed and the cartilage and bone that form the top of the nose will be shaved down with chisels. Unlike virtually all other forms of plastic surgery, a standard rhinoplasty leaves no visible scars. All of the work is internal.

Cunningham's pleasure with a challenging rhinoplasty is palpable. He bounces around the operating room, hums to himself as he inspects his tools, chats with nurses and surgical techs and the patient.

"How's it going? Can you believe this cold? This is cold for this time of year, huh?"

The patient had begun receiving sedation through an intravenous hookup, and her eyelids twitched as Cunningham rambled on and simultaneously drew several quick guidelines on her nose with a green surgical marker. She was dark-haired and olive-skinned, with high, fine cheekbones. Her nose had a thick, obvious outward bow that did not fit with her delicate face.

"What size needle do we have—can we get a twenty-seven [gauge] or a thirty?" Cunningham asked a circulating nurse, looking over his shoulder.

"I think so. Let me look," she said.

"I don't like these twenty-fives, they're too big," he said.

The nurse left and returned a minute later.

"I got these long twenty-sevens," she said.

"Perfect. Just what I wanted," Cunningham said.

He began the operation by pulling the nostril open with a small retractor called a hook and injecting an anesthetic solution into the patient's nose. The anesthetic contained the chemical epinephrine, which causes temporary constriction of the blood vessels and reduces blood loss. Cocaine is also used in rhinoplasties as an extremely efficient topical anesthetic that also has the vasculoconstrictor effect. "It's good," Cunningham said, "one of the best [anesthetics] around, but you're seeing a lot less of it because everybody's so afraid of cocaine abuse. We've got to fill out an ocean of paperwork just to get medical cocaine. And if you slip up on the paperwork, you could be in serious trouble. It's so much of a hassle that most of us have just moved on to something else. It's a shame, because it is a useful drug."

The injections continued for several minutes. Cunningham filled and refilled the syringe from a stainless-steel cup half full of anesthetic. When he was done, a resident, who would assist in the operation, washed the woman's face with pink antiseptic soap while Cunningham went out to scrub.

"We've got a couple things going on here," Cunningham said when he returned. The surgical tech was holding Cunningham's operating gown open, and he slipped his arms down the sleeves and she pulled it up over his shoulders. "She wants to lose the hump and take some of the width out of the top, but she's also had trouble breathing through one nostril. That's probably caused by allergies. So what we'll do is take out a piece of the septum [the cartilage that separates the two nostrils] and that should free up her breathing."

"You mean, she'll just have one big nasal passage inside?" blurted an observer.

"No, no, the nostrils will still be separated by the skin, there just won't be any cartilage in there, in one small spot."

"What's this going to do to the sense of smell?"

"Nothing at all. The sense of smell is located way up near the base of the brain. We don't get near it with a rhinoplasty."

With Cunningham in the gown, the tech ripped open a package of sterile rubber surgical gloves and held them so he could push his hands into them. When he was satisfied with the fit, he moved over to the patient and examined her nose. He could tell by the pale color that the epinephrine had begun to take effect. Using a pair of forceps, he soaked several gauze pads in saline solution and pushed them deep into the woman's nasal passages so she could not inhale or swallow blood during the operation. Then he looked over the tool tray and picked up a small, two-pronged hook and a scalpel. The scalpel had a blade much like a standard X-acto knife, but only about half the size.

Using the hook to grab the edge of one nostril, he pulled the nostril open and made the first careful incision just inside it.

"You've got that cartilage that makes up [the wings] of the nose, the idea is to pull it right out of there, hook it out, and cut it down a bit," Cunningham said as he worked. He switched to a pair of small scissors and continued cutting.

The anesthesiologist, who had been checking the monitors on the woman, leaned over the top of the table and asked the patient, "Can you hear me, Emily? Emily, are you okay?"

The woman muttered something that sounded like "Yes," and the anesthesiologist retreated to his chair again.

After a few minutes' work, Cunningham freed the cartilage and hooked it outside the nose. The cartilage came out as a loop about the size of a cigar band. He pushed a small hemostat through the loop to pin it fully outside the nostril. Using the scalpel and a variety of small rasps, he reshaped it, making it narrower.

That done, he repeated the procedure on the other nostril.

"A lot of the trick in plastic surgery, when you're working on two sides of anything, two nostrils or two breasts, is getting them to look alike," Cunningham said. "I remember once when I was in med school there was a case where a woman's breasts came out looking cross-eyed. A jury gave her a zillion dollars or something. You've got to get it right."

When the cartilage from the wings of the nose had been trimmed, it was allowed to slip back inside and was prodded into place.

Next, going back to a hook and scalpel, Cunningham pulled open a nostril and probed the septum until he had isolated the portion he wanted to remove. The septum, which is flexible cartilage, had bowed sideways and restricted the patient's breathing through one nostril.

Going into the nostril on the side of the bow, Cunningham made a short incision through the lining of the nose and carefully cut around the bowed-out cartilage. The piece of the septum he finally extracted was the size and shape of a crescent moon cut from a nickel. Lying on a surgical towel, it looked like a small piece of milk-jug plastic.

The operation had become bloody and the surgical tech began sucking blood from the wound with a small vacuum. Cunningham made yet another small incision just inside the nostril, and reached for a chisel. This would be the most dramatic part of the operation, the removal of the hump on the patient's nose.

"What we want to do is line the chisel up with the top of the nose, just that sliver of hump you want to remove, and then very, very carefully chisel it right out of there," Cunningham said.

Using the chisel almost like a probe, he slipped it through the incision in the nostril lining and worked it to the top of the flexible septum. Sliding it along the septum, he pushed it up the nose. He kept one hand on the chisel and the other on the ridge of the nose so he could feel the instrument's precise internal location. When he was satisfied, he thrust the chisel tip gently into the bone to create a small starting slot at the base of the hump. The resident, in the meantime, picked up a small stainless-steel surgical hammer.

"Okay," Cunningham said, when he was sure the chisel was properly placed. "Give it a couple of taps."

Tap-tap.

"A little harder."

Tap-tap.

"Uh-huh."

Tap-tap.

"And again."

Tap-tap.

"One of the guys I trained with, when he was doing one of these or a breast reduction, you'd come into the room and he'd say, 'Sorry, I can't talk now, I'm sculpting.' Pretty pretentious, huh?"

Cunningham guided the chisel up the top of the nose, taking

the nose hump off just like a skilled woodworker would take a splinter off the back of a chair. When it was done, the loose sliver of bone was removed with a small forceps.

"Now the problem is, we've taken the top off the bone, which is good, but the top [of the nose] is too wide. To fix that, we have to break her nose," he said.

That was exactly what he did.

The nasal bones extend only a short distance down the nose. If you start right between your eyes, and with your fingers slowly squeeze down the sides of the nose until suddenly the flesh collapses, you have found the ends of the nasal bones.

Normally, the nasal bones form a structure shaped like a pup tent, starting at the skull and running down to that point where the flesh collapses.

In doing the rhinoplasty, Cunningham cut the ridge line off the pup tent. Since the bones are rigid, however, they do not automatically fold together to make a nice narrow top, but must be pressed together. To get them to stay there, the bones have to be broken and rehealed in the new position.

"Have we got that hot water going?" Cunningham asked a circulating nurse.

"I'll go see."

"It was a teapot or something," Cunningham said.

"Right." The nurse left the room for the teapot.

The patient was still sleeping soundly. Cunningham used the chisel to weaken the bases of the nose bones between the eyes, then placed a thumb on one side of her nose and pressed. Hard. Nothing happened. He pressed harder, and suddenly the bone broke with a crack that raised goose bumps on an observer.

"You don't want to break it completely free. You just want to crack it on both sides, then push it together and hold it there with a splint while it heals. That gives you the nice narrow top you've been looking for," he said. And, he added, as he broke the other side, the bleeding at the site of the broken bones is mostly responsible for the black eyes that go with a nose job.

With the bones cracked and ready to be splinted, Cunningham

sewed up the several internal incisions with a small, hook-shaped needle. The nose had started to swell, but already it looked markedly different from the beginning of the operation, with a smooth, more delicate profile.

The nurse came back with a pot of hot water.

"It's really hot," she said. "Watch your fingers."

Cunningham found a square of thin white plastic on the tool table and, using a pair of surgical scissors, trimmed it into a rough triangle and dropped it into the water.

"See this? This is a splint," he said. He let it cook for a moment, retrieved it with a pair of small forceps, let it cool a bit, and then molded it over the woman's nose.

"This is really high-tech," he said with mild sarcasm. "I used to use plaster."

The splint was taped into place.

"Okay," he said after a couple of minutes of fiddling with it. Cunningham asked the nurse for a single sterile latex surgical glove. When she handed it to him, he cut off the index and middle fingers, leaving them joined with a strip of the palm. Leaning over the patient, he carefully removed the surgical sponges he'd earlier placed deep in the nasal cavities. Then he pushed one finger of the cut glove into the left nostril, and the other finger into the right nostril. The strip of latex cut from the palm still connected the fingers outside and below the nose.

"This will wick fluid out of the nose onto a four-by-four [gauze pad]," he said. He wrapped the bottom of the woman's nose with a pad and taped it into place. "This only stays on until tomorrow."

The swelling around the nose would take longer to go away. She would be back to normal "in a couple of weeks or so," although there might be subtle changes in the nose for several months, as final healing progressed.

He leaned over the woman again and raised his voice.

"Emily, we're all done, okay? It went fine, okay?"

She nodded drowsily. Cunningham gave orders to the circulating nurse that the woman's head be kept elevated, and ice packs applied around the nose to reduce swelling. He said he would check her the next day.

"That was fun, wasn't that fun?" he asked as he walked out of the room. "She's going to look good. She's going to look terrific."

The operation had taken an hour and a half. When he walked out of the room, he left behind on a surgical towel a sliver of bone, a crescent of septal cartilage, and a few stains where he wiped the rasps he used to shape the cartilages of the tip. The total mass removed from the nose would amount to less than the mass of a big toenail. But the effect on the nose was dramatic, altering the whole cast of the woman's face.

When asked if he doesn't get bored doing rhinoplasties—he does dozens of them every year—Cunningham looks faintly mystified. Why would he get bored? They are interesting operations, he says, and each one is very different. Each is an opportunity to explore the art of making beauty, of matching nose with face to make a beautiful whole.

Most of the time, he does it very well. Sometimes, he does it brilliantly. But not always.

On another day, with another patient, things did not go so well. The patient had a bulbous nose with hardly any bridge. Cunningham proposed to reshape the tip and wings of the nose and to bury some of the skin removed from the wings under the skin of the bridge, to build the bridge up.

The work went slowly as he shaped and checked, shaped and checked. Toward the end of the operation, his answers to questions and comments from the nursing staff grew terser. He said once he should be finished in ten minutes, but twenty minutes later was still working on the nose. And it was another twenty minutes before he placed the cast and pronounced it done. On the way out of the operating room, he stripped off his surgical gown and slammed it into a waste barrel.

"I couldn't do what I wanted with it. I got involved in too many compromises. You can see where you want to go, but the nose won't allow you to do it," he said as he changed clothes in the locker room.

What does that mean for the patient?

"Oh, she'll have a nice enough nose. You saw what she started with, and now she'll look pretty good. But I sit here and think that maybe she'll look in the mirror sometimes and wonder, Why couldn't I have a nose like a model? What I gave her is just kind of a nose-nose. It's all right. It's not great. I don't think I could have gotten it any better technically. It just wasn't there to work with. But I could *see* it. I could see the perfect nose for her, and I couldn't get to it."

The patient, as it happened, was quite pleased with the result. Unburdened with what might have been, she was happy with what she got. Most people are. They don't want wonderful noses. They want noses that fit.

A pretty, forty-year-old woman from Eau Claire, Wisconsin, was among those who were pleased with the outcome of her rhinoplasty.

"My biggest problem was finding a plastic surgeon. There wasn't one in our town until recently, and I didn't know anybody who'd gone outside for surgery. I didn't want to trust my face to just anybody. Then I read about Cunningham and decided he was the guy for me," Kelly said.

Kelly first heard comments about her nose in elementary school: "It was about fifth grade, someone mentioned they liked my Roman nose. That's when I became aware that I didn't have a little turned-up pug nose like everybody else. People have always told me that I was pretty, but other people made cruel comments, I guess, and that made me self-conscious."

She was so self-conscious that she didn't like photos taken from the side, and was wary of any light that might emphasize her nose. Her husband, she said, "liked me like I was, but he said if I wanted surgery, that was fine. He just said he didn't want me changed, he didn't want me to look a lot different, because he did like me."

She was apprehensive before the surgery "because I didn't want to look like somebody else. Dr. Cunningham said I wouldn't, but I was a little worried anyway. We had a long talk, and I told him that I wanted the smallest nose I could get that still fit with my face."

Cunningham said that nothing radical would be done.

"I finally decided to leave it up to him. He said he had to work with what was already there, just like when you're remodeling a house. Or in my case, an eight-plex," she said wryly.

Her rhinoplasty was done under sedation, rather than general anesthetic. She woke up at one point, while Cunningham was breaking her nose bones to narrow the top.

"It didn't hurt. It just felt a little uncomfortable. In fact, my nose never really hurt after the operation. The worst thing was that I couldn't blow my nose. I have allergies, and felt really stuffed up for a while, and that was uncomfortable.

"Dr. Cunningham said I'd have black eyes, and I'd read some articles and figured I might have black eyes for six weeks. I went out looking for cosmetics to cover it up if I could. It turned out that the black eyes were gone in two weeks. I went to see my family doctor in three weeks, and he said, 'Your nose looks wonderful, but where are the black-and-blue marks?' "

The nose, she said, was exactly what she had been looking for.

"I have a nice nose, but it's not something I think about anymore. It fits. It's not a factor for me now. A few weeks after the operation I went visiting family all over the state, and we hadn't told people, and they all said, 'You know, you look different, but I don't know what it is.' That was just perfect for me. My mother knew about the operation. She drove all the way down from Wausau to look at it, and she thought it made a big difference. But then, she was looking for the change."

Kelly's biggest regret is that she didn't have the rhinoplasty sooner. She recommends the operation to any young girl who feels self-conscious about a large nose.

"I have a friend who had what they call 'car door' ears. When she was about nine the other kids were really cruel about it. Finally her family decided to do something about it, and she had surgery. It changed her life completely. That's what can happen."

Snapshot: Anesthesia

When a general anesthetic hits a patient, the transformation is dramatic. The patient falls from a nervous watchfulness to unconsciousness in a matter of seconds. The face and jaw go slack, the eyes roll up, the entire body relaxes.

At the deepest stages of general anesthesia, the body can be manipulated like a sack of laundry without fear of physical resistance or psychological trauma.

Anesthesia is a complicated matter. If not done with care, it could cause a patient to drop straight through full anesthesia into coma and death. It is a field for specialists.

Anesthesia is usually induced by an anesthesiologist. When the patient is asleep and stable, he turns the monitoring of the operation over to a nurse-anesthetist. The anesthesiologist frequently covers several operations simultaneously, periodically checking with each nurse-anesthetist. He returns at the end of each operation to supervise the lifting of anesthesia.

The anesthesiologist and the nurse-anesthetist sit at the end of the operating table, by the patient's head, surrounded by monitoring equipment. It is their job to keep track of the patient's vital signs and to regulate fluids and anesthetic drugs used during the operation. Either a nurse-anesthetist or an anesthesiologist is present for every moment of an operation.

Anesthesia is no longer a matter of slapping an ether-soaked mask over the patient's face. An anesthesiologist uses a variety of drugs—ether rarely is used anymore—chosen for various characteristics needed for a particular operation or patient.

The purpose of anesthesia, of course, is to render a patient insensible to pain. That can be done in several ways. The anesthetic block may be local, as with a dental injection that numbs a tooth. It may be regional, as with a spinal injection that blocks pain in the legs. Or it may be general, rendering the patient unconscious.

In discussing general anesthesia, Dr. Paul Molinari, an anesthesiologist at St. Paul–Ramsey Medical Center, said there are three practical planes of consciousness: stage one, the waking state; stage two, a dangerous intermediate state; and stage three, the surgical level of general anesthesia.

"You want to take a person from the waking state down to stage three as quickly as you safely can," Molinari said. "When the patient's awake, he can control himself, and when he's in stage three, we can control him. But in stage two, he can create problems for himself. He might thrash around, cough, or vomit and obstruct his airway. . . . We try to get through it quickly."

Patients on an operating table usually look as if they are under general anesthetic. More and more often, they are not. Instead, they are heavily sedated to relax them, and a local anesthetic is used to kill the pain of the operation. The two—general anesthetic and heavy sedation—are often confused, but are radically different.

In anesthesia, pain signals do not register with the brain as pain. With sedation, which is akin to sleep, they do.

"If you pinch somebody who is asleep, they feel it. If you do it hard enough, they wake up," Molinari said. "You could sedate somebody so heavily that he couldn't wake up, but the pain would still be registering, just as if he were asleep. His blood pressure would go out of sight, his heart would start pounding. With anesthesia, the pain literally doesn't register, and you don't get those effects."

Much plastic surgery is done with sedation and local anesthesia. The sedation relaxes the patient, or even puts her to sleep, while the local blocks the pain. Dentists do the same thing when they give a nervous patient nitrous oxide (laughing gas) as a relaxant and then inject a local anesthetic to numb the tooth.

Sedation with a local anesthetic is often preferred over general anesthesia because general anesthesia is riskier. A certain tiny percentage of patients are killed by the anesthesia itself. Other people may suffer unpleasant side effects, such as several hours of nausea. About 1 percent of patients who have had general anesthesia suffer nausea for eight hours or more.

Those unpleasant side effects are largely absent with sedation, although some patients still experience episodes of nausea.

Because sedation only relaxes, while the local anesthetic is used to kill the pain, plastic surgery patients are often functionally awake. That is true even with relatively complicated surgery such as facelifts, rhinoplasties, and breast implants.

A number of plastic-surgery patients interviewed for this book could recall operating-room conversations after the operation. Some hospitals routinely put signs on operating room doors to warn newcomers to the room that the "Patient Is Awake."

"That's to keep some guy from coming in and blurting out, you know, 'My God, what have you done to the poor guy,'" Cunningham said. "Just kidding around, you could scare the brains out of somebody."

Once, during a suction lipectomy, two nurses were talking about the operation, and one told the other that she had had a lipectomy herself, with a different surgeon, and that she was pleased with the result.

"It really hurt, though. I was black and blue like somebody beat me up with a softball bat, or something. I really looked gross," she said.

"Will somebody get her outa here?" Cunningham said in a joking voice that carried an undertone of warning. The conversation resumed outside the operating room. The patient had been given general anesthesia, but Cunningham said later it's good policy to stay away from that kind of talk.

"You have to be particularly careful when you're working with a resident and you're showing him how to do something. If the patient is awake, she might not understand what's happening," he said.

On the other hand, most anesthetic and sedative drugs create a certain level of amnesia. That is desirable.

"Sometimes when you're working [with a local anesthetic and sedation] you'll do something that hurts—it usually happens at the end of an operation when the effects of the drug might be wearing off a bit. You haven't put in any more because we're wary of putting in any more drugs than we're sure we need. So maybe you snip a flap of skin or put in a stitch and the patient flinches or even says something to you . . . so then we put in more anesthetic.

"But the quality of forgetfulness—she won't remember when she wakes up—is important. When she does wake up, there won't be any psychological problems with pain or fear of operations. . . . There just won't be anything there, at least not with minor pain."

Aside from the rare emergencies involving anesthetics, the most common problem they cause involves the depth to which the patient relaxes. Once a patient is fully relaxed, she is extremely difficult to manipulate. Her arms, legs, and head would flop wildly if not carefully handled. And because the patient is so floppy, there is a tendency to grab and squeeze. That can lead to bruises and other damage.

The recovery period for modern anesthetics is short.

"We don't want a slow recovery for the same reason we don't want a slow induction. We want to minimize the period when nobody has control over the patient's actions," Molinari said.

Even though the recovery is quick, there will be some lingering effects.

"We don't suggest you have your rhinoplasty and jump in the car and drive home," Cunningham said. "You'd wind up wrapped around a phone pole."

Breasts

A YOUNG blonde woman removed her hospital top and sat on the edge of an examining table, nude to the waist, as Cunningham gave her a last brief check. In a few moments, she would ride a gurney down to the operating room for a breast enhancement.

The woman was stunning—lithe, athletic, with sun-bleached hair, green eyes, clear skin, and high, fine cheekbones. Her breasts were small, but there was nothing unfeminine about her body. She had agreed to allow the author to follow her through the procedure (as did all the patients reported in this book), and now, as she sat with her top off, I confess to small shock.

Of her type, which might be thought of as athletic Scandinavian, she seemed nearly perfect. Granted that Cunningham is a highly skilled surgeon, why would she do this? Why would she do anything? Almost any change, it seemed to the author, would be a loss.

And that is a reflection of the complexity of the issues involved in breast enhancements. The author has always found small-breasted, athletic women to be particularly attractive. Other men have suggested to him that small-breasted women are the unfortunate victims of an unhappy fate, doomed to go through life with a serious disfigurement.

The same feelings seem to be held by women: some small-breasted women feel sorely afflicted and would hock the ranch for larger breasts. On the other hand, some women with very large breasts would do almost anything to be smaller. . . .

Breast operations are unquestionably among the most psychologically complex aesthetic works of a plastic surgeon. Breasts are the focus of critical issues—beauty, femininity, motherhood, sexuality, personal identity, and relationships with others. Changes in the breasts can have profound impact on both patients and their mates.

It is an area that is difficult to discuss without risking charges of sexist impulses and unhealthy fixations.

Whatever arguments might be made about the *why* of breast operations, Cunningham argues that most women who inquire about aesthetic breast changes want the work done for themselves, from their own inner needs, as a result of their own sense of personal image.

A few, of course, do not.

A few are having it done to satisfy the desires of somebody else—a mate or a parent. In those cases, if Cunningham cannot satisfy himself that the patient has a personal desire for the change, he will "suggest another opinion." That's doctor talk that means he won't do the work.

(The problem is more complicated than it seems. Some women are embarrassed by their dissatisfaction with their breasts. They may suggest that they are "doing this" for someone else, when the someone else may be perfectly satisfied with the patient's breasts. It may take extended consultation to sort it all out.)

Cunningham is also wary of the woman who is vague about her goals. She wants her breasts changed, but can't clearly state what is wrong with them as they are. Nor can she say exactly what she wants. Sometimes the patient is simply inarticulate. Others are looking for a surgical solution for social and psychological problems. Breast surgery almost certainly isn't their answer.

Most patients, fortunately, are not like that. Most are clear about their goals. They shop for skill and price, and are quite blunt in their investigations. One young woman, a candidate for breast enhancement, showed up at Cunningham's office with a selection of breast samples culled from *Playboy* magazine. She could illustrate with blueprint precision exactly what she had in mind.

"That can be a drawback, too," Cunningham said. "Sometimes there are places you just can't go, given what you're starting with. Part of the job is to point out the limitations."

While a good plastic surgeon can generally promise aesthetically excellent breasts, he may not be able to promise precisely the breasts of a particular model.

The four most common breast operations are the *enhancement*, which makes small breasts larger; the *breast reduction*, which makes overly large breasts smaller; the *mastopexy*, which lifts, shapes, and tightens drooping breasts; and the *breast reconstruction*, for women who have undergone cancer-related mastectomies (breast removals). Reconstructions will be treated in a later chapter.

Of all the operations done by plastic surgeons, the breast enhancement, technically called an augmentation mammoplasty, is the most like magic. The change in the body is immediate and dramatic and generally unobscured by the bruising and unsightly sutures left by most surgery.

Before a breast enhancement, Cunningham consults with the patient to determine the suitability of surgery. Once he accepts a patient, they together determine about what size breasts she should have. Most women opt for breasts that are moderately large for their body size, expressed as a full-B or small-C brassiere cup. Women who have later operations that provide an opportunity to change breast size almost always stay with the initial choice of moderately large breasts.

To determine exactly what the patient has in mind, Cunningham may suggest that she buy a brassiere of a particular size, fill it out with paper padding, and then put on a blouse or a sweater "to see if the image she gets is the one she wants."

Once all of that is determined, an operating date is set.

. . .

One enhancement operation began with the patient scrubbed and sedated on the operating table, but still able to talk with the surgical team. The nurses covered her with sterile blue drapes, leaving only the chest area exposed.

The woman's breast circumference was average, but her breasts were very thin—not much thicker than her hand. They looked as though tea saucers had been inverted and placed under her chest skin. Her nipples were fully developed.

When Cunningham was ready to begin work, the anesthesiologist injected a measured pulse of anesthetic into an IV tube that led down to her arm. The clear liquid drained down through the tube, and in a moment, the patient was sleeping soundly. When she was stable, Cunningham injected local anesthetics into the breasts using a large syringe with a long needle. The procedure took several minutes and is unpleasant to watch, though the patient seemed unaware of it. The injections were doing double duty: in addition to the pain blocker, the anesthetic fluid contained epinephrine to close down blood vessels and help limit bleeding during the operation.

"Okay, you see how the [pink] color [of the breasts] changes as the epinephrine goes in, they get paler? That's what we're looking for," Cunningham said. He waited a few minutes, checked the tool kit a last time, looked at the breasts again, and said, "Knife."

The surgical tech handed him a scalpel. Using one hand to move the bulk of the breast up a bit, Cunningham made a short incision, about two inches long. The incision was made where the new, larger breast would fold down. The scar would fit into the fold and be practically invisible after healing.

Using a cautery, scissors, and a scalpel to separate the fat and glandular tissue of the breast from the underlying muscle, Cunningham began to tunnel beneath the breast. The idea is to separate the tissue that makes up the mass of the breast from the tissue tied to the rib cage. The result is a narrow opening where the incision is made, which then spreads beneath the surface of the whole mass of the breast. Two people are needed for the work. The resident retracts, lifting the breast and chest tissue away from the rib cage with a large, L-shaped fiber-optic retractor. The surgeon works with his scalpel, scissors, and cautery. The fiber optic illuminates the excavation so the surgeon can see what he is doing.

It took fifteen or twenty minutes for Cunningham to open a pocket approximately the size needed. That done, he exchanged the scalpel for a cautery and spent a couple of minutes locating and cauterizing small bleeders.

"Is that test implant ready?" he asked the tech.

"Sure is." She turned and picked up the implant and held it out to him.

Breast implants are tough, pliable plastic bags filled with liquid silicone, about the size and shape of a small hamburger bun. Both the skin of the plastic bag and the silicone are crystal clear, and handling them is like handling a fist-sized drop of magically cohesive water. The bags feel almost, but not quite, like flesh. They are not required to feel exactly like flesh because real breast tissue will lie above them when the surgery is complete.

Implants come in several sizes. Experienced plastic surgeons can closely judge the sizes needed, but two or three are usually tried before a decision is made.

Taking the test implant from the surgical tech, Cunningham compressed it to fit through the small incision and slipped it beneath the breast tissue. After manipulating it for a moment to get it precisely in place, he stepped back for a better perspective on it. The woman's breast looked completely natural, and very well shaped, but substantially larger. Cunningham turned to the resident who was assisting with the operation.

"What do you think, is that too big?" he asked.

"Well, I'd say that's a C for sure," the resident replied.

"Let's try another one."

Cunningham squeezed the first test implant out of the pocket and put in a second, smaller one. The size difference was immediately apparent.

"Gee, I don't know," said the resident. "If she wanted to be in the B-C area, that might be a little small."

"You think so?"

Cunningham was already taking the second test implant out. He slipped the first one back in and stepped away from the table. "Hmm. I think this is the one. Looks pretty good, huh?" He was looking at a nurse.

She shrugged: "Yeah, looks pretty good to me."

"Okay." Cunningham looked pleased. "It looks really good."

He took the test implant out and lifted the breast again, peering into the excavated area with the fiber-optic light. "I think we want . . . ," he muttered to himself. He picked up a scalpel and cut a little further under the breast. The patient suddenly stirred and opened her eyes.

"When are we going to start?" she asked sleepily.

"We already started," said the nurse-anesthetist.

"When?"

"You went to sleep for a while there, and we put the local anesthetic in," Cunningham said.

Cunningham began cauterizing bleeders with the electric cautery. "What are you doing now?" the patient asked as the cautery's monitor beeped.

"We're using a special machine to lift the breast tissue to make space."

"Well, if you find a couple of extra . . ." She seemed to doze off in midsentence.

"Extra what?" Cunningham prompted.

Pause. "I don't know. . . ." She giggled and was asleep again.

A few minutes later she roused herself and said, "Will they always be like this or will I have to come in and have something done to them?"

"No, no, there's no maintenance," Cunningham said. "It'd be a real drag if you had to come in every twelve thousand miles and have them rotated, wouldn't it?"

She giggled again and went back to sleep. Cunningham finished the excavation and slipped the larger of the two test implants back under the breast.

"That looks better," he said to the resident. "You want the test implant to make the breast look a little bigger than you actually want it to be." He explained that test implants have thicker and less flexible plastic skins than the real ones. Given two implants of the same volume, the test implant will push the breast out farther.

"If you put in a test implant and it looks perfect, the real implant will [make the breast] come out a little small. If the test implant looks a little big, it should be just right," he said.

He removed the test implant a final time and began work on the second breast. After trying two different test implants on the second side, he was satisfied with that excavation and asked for the actual implants.

A nurse produced a sealed sterile package and opened it, letting the surgical tech lift the implant from the package. She handed it to Cunningham, who dipped it in sterile saline solution to make it slippery and easier to manipulate. He folded it a bit and pushed it into place. After another check to make sure the position was correct, he carefully and quickly sewed up the incision.

The procedure was repeated on the other side. This time, the size problem could have been more difficult—not only does the surgeon have to make the breast larger, it must match the other side. In this particular case, the match was not difficult.

(Matching breast sizes becomes a matter of central concern in another kind of breast-enhancement operation, one that is done not to make both breasts larger, but to make one the same size as the other. Most women have slightly different-sized or different-shaped breasts, but usually the difference is so small as to be unnoticeable. It remains a personal idiosyncrasy, rather than a disfiguration. In a few cases, however, there is a gross disparity in sizes, which can be corrected with an enhancement. Even in those cases, though, the enhancement is usually bilateral. One breast is made substantially larger, the other a bit larger to match.)

As Cunningham worked on closing the second incision, the talk suddenly jumped to movies. Cunningham is an avid movie fan.

"What's the word on the street about *Heartburn?*" he asked. The resident said he hadn't seen it.

"I'd give money that Meryl Streep has had a rhinoplasty," Cunningham said. "It looks too trim."

That observation led to a general discussion of Mariel Hemingway's breast enhancement:

"I saw her in *Personal Best* and her breasts are almost child-like, preadolescent," said one of the operating-room staffers.

"You get to *Star 80* and it's all changed. I guess she had to do it for the part, the Playboy bunny part," Cunningham said. "Looked like a pretty good job."

He added that a lot of women athletes have breast implants, as Hemingway did after *Personal Best*, in which she played the part of an Olympic-class hurdler.

"You get a top athlete, they're carrying almost no body fat. There's just nothing there, and they start feeling self-conscious about their breasts. When we do the implants on them, they look terrific. As a general rule, you don't get slobs coming in for implants. They're very attractive women."

When Cunningham finished suturing the second incision, the nurses began tearing down the sterile coverings on and around the operating table. The patient woke again, quickly becoming more alert than at any time since the operation began. Cunningham wanted her a bit more upright, so he could properly position some pads under her breasts. As a nurse helped her sit up, the woman looked down at herself.

"Wow," she said, and smiled.

Later, when the woman had been taken to a recovery room, Cunningham was asked what would happen if she were hit hard in the breasts.

"It would be possible to burst one of the pads, but it would take something really hard, like an automobile accident where your ribs are broken. Even with an injury, the fluid wouldn't go anywhere—the body reacts to it in a very neutral way. It doesn't pass it on to the brain, or anything. You'd just take it out and put in a new pad."

He added that scar tissue forms all around the excavation, and would eventually hold the implants very firmly in place.

There are a number of myths surrounding breast-implant operations. One, that the breast pad can somehow "melt" and then "reharden," leaving the victim with permanently misshapen breasts, is defeated by the simple fact that the silicone pads aren't hard in the first place.

Another myth says that changes in pressure (as from going up in an airplane, or down in scuba gear) may cause the implants to explode. That doesn't happen. Ever.

"The biggest problem we have is capsulization, where scar tissue forms around the implants and begins tightening down too much. That squeezes the pads, and you can get a tennis ball effect. If that happens, sometimes we have to go back in and release the scar tissue," Cunningham said. He estimated that 10 to 15 percent of breast-enhancement patients encounter capsulization problems to a greater or lesser degree. You can reduce the chance of it by massaging the breasts for five minutes a day until they're healed, to keep down the rigidity of the scar tissue.

"There aren't many other adverse effects—her nerves are fine, and she still has full sensitivity in her nipples and skin. A lover could manipulate her breasts any way he wanted without endangering the viability of the implant. It's really a pretty clean operation," he said.

Later he was asked about the sexist implications of breast-enhancement operations. Small, flat breasts generally have no functional problems—they are as efficient at nursing as larger breasts—so enhancements are purely cosmetic operations.

"I've heard people suggest that operations like breast enhancements are somehow sexist, sure. You know that they wouldn't be undergoing this pain and trauma if it weren't for men and their fixations. But I don't give that much credence," Cunningham said. "A lot of these operations, maybe sixty percent, are done on women who have had children. During the period when they were lactating, their breasts got much larger. And then when they stopped lactating, they got smaller again.

Sometimes, they get smaller than they were before the pregnancy, and then they're stuck with this shriveled-up skin, too. Most women aren't fixed on the idea of large sexy breasts. They want to look like they did before the pregnancy, what they always were and what they were comfortable with.

"So are they doing it for men or are they doing it for themselves? I think they're doing it for themselves. I don't think there's anything particularly sexist about trying to look good."

What about those women who simply want to be bigger—who don't have the problems associated with pregnancy?

"There is a sexual identity, an image of femininity that most women look for. Like adolescent boys might look for beard development, adolescent girls look for breast development. If it doesn't happen, they may have this sense of something missing. Again, I don't think there's anything particularly sexist about it. It's reality. If a woman has a strong sense of something missing, and she can change it, why not do it?"

Large numbers of American women apparently agree with that sentiment. About 94,000 breast augmentations were done in 1986 by board-certified plastic surgeons, making it the second most popular aesthetic operation after suction lipectomies.

Two other aesthetic breast operations, reductions and mastopexies (the breast lifting and shaping operations), are similar to each other, and are much less clean than enhancements—there's more fluid loss involved and more chance of nerve damage. Damage to glandular tissue may make it impossible for the woman to nurse a baby.

"We used to tell patients that they'd automatically lose the ability to nurse, but we find that it's not quite as automatic as we thought," Cunningham said. "Lots of them find that they can still nurse, but some still lose it. So we tell patients that they have to count on losing it. If they don't, then that's a bonus."

These operations also involve some visible scarring, but the majority of breast-reduction candidates are willing to accept the scarring in exchange for smaller breasts. While women who get breast enhancements do so for aesthetic and psychological reasons, breast reduction patients actually feel physically handicapped by their large breast size. Most have not been able to run, or to participate in any sports that require running, since their early teenage years. Often, they are victims of teasing by other women and of unwelcome sexual comments and attention from men, which make them painfully self-conscious. Consequently, they look upon their large breasts as a curse, a disease. A few scars are a small price to pay to be rid of them.

One of Cunningham's reduction patients was a young actress with very large, somewhat pendulous breasts who found their size to be a disadvantage in dancing and other acrobatic activities.

Cunningham and a resident met the woman in the prep room and began by asking her to open her hospital gown so Cunningham could mark her breasts with a surgical pen.

The first line through each breast, running vertically through the nipple, would help in the relocation of the nipple "up higher on the same line, and just over the inframammary fold," Cunningham said. He turned to the resident: "If there's a question in your mind about whether to put it on X or Y, put it on the lower one. If there's a problem, you've got something left to work with. Give yourself some leeway."

Taking a small metal ruler from his pocket, Cunningham carefully drew a triangle on each breast, with the apex just above the nipple. That, he said, was the general area from which the tissue would be removed.

When he was finished with his marking, the patient was taken on a gurney to the operating room, to be prepped for the operation, and Cunningham went down to the lunchroom for a quick snack. Fifteen minutes later, after eating a package of cookies and scrubbing, he arrived in the operating room and found everybody ready but the anesthesiologist, who was out on a different case.

Cunningham was irritated and told the nurse, "Don't start the clock on this thing. We're not going to charge her for using the operating room when we're all just standing around."

The nurse nodded, said "Okay," and made a note on a chart. The anesthesiologist showed up five minutes later, apologized, and said he had been starting another case.

He checked the patient and then took her down. When she was unconscious, he inserted a breathing tube in her throat, taped her eyes, and padded her elbows "because the way she's lying she could get a lot of pressure on the nerves in those areas and we don't want to mess up her hand control."

When the anesthesiologist finished his work, the resident began scrubbing the woman's breasts, upper chest, and abdomen with antiseptic soap, a process that took five minutes. When he finished, Cunningham and the surgical technician, both in sterile gowns by now, covered the woman with sterile sheets, leaving exposed only a rectangle over her breasts. The scrubbing had blurred the guidelines on the patient's breasts, and before going to work, Cunningham quickly sketched them back in with a sterile surgical marker.

"Breasts sag and flatten differently when she's lying on her back than when she's upright, and that's why we draw on her when she's awake and sitting up," Cunningham said. After redrawing the faded lines, he picked up a glass, much like a shot glass, centered it on her nipple, and drew around it. The resulting circle neatly paralleled the edge of the areola around the nipple. Then he drew another, identical circle farther up the centering line he'd drawn earlier.

"The idea is, we cut out the nipple but we leave a stalk beneath it, with its nerves and blood vessels intact. Then we take out the tissue, excavate that circle [the one farther up the breast] and reinsert the nipple in there. That gives you a much smaller breast and higher nipple complex."

When the nipple is cut out so precisely, Cunningham said, "You do get something of a bull's-eye effect" because the procedure eliminates the usual fading between the areola and the surrounding breast skin. The "bull's-eye effect" will diminish in time be-

cause of what is usually thought of as a liability in plastic surgery—
the scarring.

"The scar will actually add a fading effect," Cunningham said.
"The final result is usually pretty good."

In some candidates for breast reductions, the unusual growth
of their breasts also causes the darker skin of the areola to stretch
and expand to an unpleasing degree. The "bull's-eye" created by
isolating the nipple also reduces the size of the areola, which, in
most cases, is a desired cosmetic effect.

When Cunningham was ready to begin, he looked up at the
resident, who was now dressed in a sterile gown and leaning
over the table, and said, "You have to [cut] straight down around
the pedicle [nipple stalk]. If we undermine it too much we'll cut
the blood vessels going up to the nipple."

And he demonstrated with his usual style, a precise but nonchalant initial incision with a fairly large-bladed scalpel.

A breast reduction is a bloody operation, done with the constant *zzzttt* and *beep* of the electric cautery and the smell of
burning fat and blood. The breast fat itself is not pretty: it is
contained in bulging, amber-colored, greasy-textured cells.

The operating field is a large triangle, with the point at the
top, the base at the bottom of the breast. The natural nipple is
centered just below the point. Working slowly to minimize tissue
damage, Cunningham first isolated the nipple and then cut away
the triangle-shaped chunk of fat and skin around and below it.
Altogether, he removed two fist-sized lumps of fat and dropped
them into a stainless-steel container.

When he was satisfied with the amount of fat removed from
the bottom of the breast, he moved to the top of the triangle and
the circle he'd drawn earlier. That was where the nipple stalk
would be reinserted. Carefully cutting around the circle, he created a deep, bloody "keyhole" at the top of the breast, removing
a third fist-sized chunk of fat. Below it, the nipple was isolated
on a stalk of tissue that included the nerves and blood vessels
that serviced it.

When he felt he'd removed about enough tissue, Cunningham
folded the nipple into the upper keyhole. The fit was too tight.

"That's okay, because this is where you figure what you have to do to finish it," he said to the resident. "You don't want to take too much too soon."

After manipulating the nipple stalk in and out of the keyhole in the upper breast, he cut away some more skin and fat. The final fitting took three tries. With the final trim, the breast—which moments before looked terribly mutilated—neatly folded together like a three-dimensional jigsaw puzzle. Cunningham and the resident quickly sutured the wounds.

As in all cases where the skin is cut through, there would be scars. One, located under the breast, normally would be invisible. A second scar, around the areola, eventually would resemble the normal blending between the color of the areola and the skin of the surrounding breast. The third scar would be visible. It would run vertically from the fold beneath the breast, up the front of the breast to the bottom of the areola. The vertical scar would be white, and about the thickness of a hair, although complications could produce a thicker, heavier scar.

As in most breast operations, other than those for cancer, this one was bilateral. After finishing with the first breast, Cunningham repeated the entire procedure on the second.

In few pairs of breasts are both shaped exactly alike. "Why aren't they usually the same?" Cunningham asked rhetorically as he finished the second breast. "Well, left- or right-handedness could have something to do with it, extra muscle development on one side or the other, but mostly they're just not the same."

When he finished with the second breast, Cunningham supervised the bandaging and gave instructions for the patient's overnight stay at the hospital. "She should be able to go home tomorrow," he told the resident. "Let me know if she has any problems, but it looks pretty good."

Cosmetic breast surgery can involve a painful recovery—not incapacitating pain, but certainly enough to be a factor in deciding whether to have the operation.

Carolyn, who underwent a breast-enhancement operation, said,

"I thought [the pain] wasn't supposed to be a big deal, but for me it was a big deal. It bothered me quite a bit, especially right after the operation. I had some pain off and on for about four weeks.

"The pain was not where the incision was, but inside, in the gland. I would ache, and then sometimes there would be sharp stabbing pains. Right after the operation, I could get up and move around, but I didn't want to move fast."

Carolyn also suffered hypersensitivity of the nipple. Even gentle manipulation was painful at first. Several months after the operation, her nipples were still sensitive, although she thought the sensitivity might be declining. She also thought the skin on the bottom of her breasts might be somewhat less sensitive than it had been before the operation.

Pain is difficult to describe objectively. It affects different people in different ways. Two indexes of its severity are the willingness of the patient to suffer it again, and her ability to move around or work while suffering it.

Carolyn, who found that the pain "was a big deal," qualified her statement by saying that given a choice, she would choose to have the surgery again. She said that she did, in fact, plan to have a tummy tuck with suction lipectomy on some small saddlebags on her hips, although she had been warned that the tuck and lipectomy were more painful than the breast enhancement.

Carolyn noted that she had had the surgery on a Friday, was back to work on Monday, and that the pain was not strong enough to affect her work.

"I did hunch my shoulders sometimes, and a friend said, 'What's wrong, does your back hurt?' I said, 'Oh, yes, my back hurts a little.' " She also took some painkilling drugs.

The day after the operation, Carolyn looked at herself in a mirror and was stunned. "They were huge. I thought Dr. Cunningham had made a mistake and put in the wrong size implants. But that was swelling. It went down after a while, and they were okay. Pretty big, I wear a C cup, but the appearance is very satisfying."

The scars from the incisions are about two inches long. Several months after the operation they were still red, but the redness was fading. Carolyn's breasts now fold down over the scars. She can't see the scars without lifting a breast or stretching her arms over her head and leaning back while looking in a mirror.

Carolyn is in her middle thirties. She began to worry about the small size of her breasts when she was seventeen or eighteen.

"I was absolutely flat, with a little nipple, and I thought something was wrong with me. I went to a doctor and he said nothing was wrong, it was just heredity. I wondered how it could be heredity when my mother and grandmother had such big breasts.

"Anyway, that's when it would have made sense for me to get the enhancement, but I didn't know you could do that, then. But that's when you really focus on your body and it's really important how you look," she said.

She thought about getting the enhancement for a long time before she went ahead with it. The actual decision was spurred by interest in a different cosmetic operation, a tummy tuck.

"My first baby, I didn't gain too much weight. With the second, I gained fifty-five pounds. I was out to here. There was a lot of loose skin afterward, and it bothered me. I wanted to get a tummy tuck to get rid of it. So I went to get a tummy tuck, and I asked [Cunningham] about the enhancement, and decided to go ahead with both of them. I scheduled the tummy tuck first, and then the enhancement, but when the time came for the tummy tuck, I had a crisis going on at work and I had to cancel. Everything [at work] was settled when the time came for the enhancement, so I went ahead. I still have to reschedule for the tummy tuck."

Her new breast size now feels normal, she said: "I can't remember what it was like the other way." The breasts themselves feel almost, but not quite, natural.

"I think they might be a little too firm for a woman my age. They have a firmness like you might have on a teenge girl, like a well-developed sixteen-year-old."

Overall, Carolyn said she was pleased with the decision to have the operation. She said the operation was done for herself, not for her husband—"I don't think it mattered that much to him."

"I like the way I look, but there are other things, too. I can wear brassieres. You don't know what it was like, where you'd have to look through brand after brand after brand and not find any bras that fit. They'd ride up to your neck. . . . Now I go in and get bras that fit."

The operation held one odd surprise: she seemed somewhat bemused with the cost of the implants, at $400.

"They look like little bags of water. I thought, four hundred dollars? But that's what they cost, I guess. I wouldn't want anything cheap in there."

Denise shared many of Carolyn's personal statistics. She is thirty-five, and began to worry about her breasts when she was in her teens. One big difference: Denise's were far too big, rather than too small.

"I began to develop when I was about fifteen, and then just never quit," she said. She didn't get much sympathy from her mother because her mother was small-breasted and "probably would like to be a little bigger."

There is nothing funny, she said, about being teased about the large size of your breasts.

"I had to put up with it since I was fifteen. I hated it. I could never wear what I wanted to wear, or people would stare. I always had to camouflage them. Men say the most awful things to you, it's shocking. They'd never say the same things to women with small breasts. Somehow, if you've got big breasts, they think it's okay to say anything they want," she said. "Another thing that used to drive me crazy. People, especially men, talked to your breasts. You'd be trying to have a conversation, or you'd ask a sales clerk a question, and instead of looking you in the eye, they'd look down here. It drives you crazy."

Denise is small, barely five feet, two inches tall. She wore double-D-sized brassieres. (The buyer of women's lingerie for a major department store said that double-D "isn't so much of a regular size as kind of a container. . . . I've never waited on anyone who was buying double-D-size brassieres who seemed to be proud of her breasts. They're always apologizing and they seem embarrassed. I feel sorry for them.")

Denise, even weeks after her operation, referred to her over-sized breasts as "them," as though they had been separate and somewhat unpleasant members of the family. She never considered large breasts any kind of gift.

"They were so big that my back would hurt, trying to hold up the weight. I couldn't find clothes that would fit right, I always had to wear those big floppy blouses. I had trouble with my bra straps cutting into my neck muscles. I couldn't ever run. Running was out of the question. It was like being fat, but I wasn't fat. And then there were the comments you'd hear, even from women. It was awful."

Denise's sister, who is several years younger, had the same problem.

"She was always more outgoing than I was. I was the quiet one. She didn't try to hide her breasts like I did, and she paid for it. The things people said to her were incredible. To make it worse, she worked in a bar for a while, and men she'd never seen before would come up and make all kinds of comments. I used to get mad just hearing what they'd say."

The younger sister got fed up and had a breast reduction. Denise liked the results, but was in the middle of starting a family and decided to wait before considering one for herself. Eventually, as she entered her thirties, the time came. Her husband said he liked her as she was, but would also be happy to see her get a breast reduction: he would support anything she decided to do.

Husbands are in a difficult situation when it comes to cosmetic surgery on their wives. There is no correct answer to the question, "Should I have a breast reduction?" (or enhancement, or nose job). A yes brings the follow-up question, "How long haven't you liked me the way I am?" A no means that he might not support an operation the wife desperately wants. Women who have had a cosmetic operation suggest that the question not be hinted at, or asked casually, but be approached directly: "I am thinking about having a breast reduction, something I've wanted for years. I want to talk about it." With this approach, the husband is not faced with the classic "Have you stopped beating your wife?" quandary, where any answer he gives could be misinterpreted.

"I tried to be really rational about the reduction," Denise said. "I decided to sit down and make up a list of all the good points of having big breasts. I couldn't come up with any and decided to go ahead."

She had a problem finding a doctor. "My family doctor wasn't any help at all. I think he liked them big."

She didn't want to risk a poor result, and also wanted someone who would be sympathetic to her plight. She made some preliminary inquiries with a medical referral service, but then, at a critical point in her decision process, read a newspaper article about Cunningham. A few days later, she called and made an appointment.

"My biggest fear was that he'd take one look and say, 'Aw, they're not that big, you don't need a reduction,' and I'd be stuck with them for the rest of my life. He didn't say that. Another thing was, when he talked to me, he looked at my eyes, and not at my breasts. He said my problem wasn't trivial. That decided me, and I went for the operation."

Denise had never had surgery before and found the preoperation procedures a bit frightening. Then she was on the table, and out. She didn't feel or hear a thing, and woke up with B-cup breasts.

She stayed in the hospital for two days. There was some pain, she said, but not as much as she expected. She did not take any of the pain pills prescribed for her, although she did take an aspirin on the second or third day after she got home.

A month after the operation she still felt an occasional soreness and thought she might have lost some degree of sensitivity in one nipple. The scarring from a breast reduction is significant, and not as well hidden as it is on a breast enhancement. She said the scars would not be a problem.

"I don't care about all that, the feeling and the scars. I just feel great. I went out and bought a tube top. It's like somebody all of a sudden set you free."

Members of the American Society of Plastic and Reconstructive Surgeons did about 48,600 breast reductions in 1986, up from about 37,700 in 1984 and 32,000 in 1982. The rate of growth in numbers of operations is one of the highest in the field of cosmetic surgery.

Snapshot: Wound Care

When everything is said and done, the goal of a plastic surgeon is simple: to create a well-healed wound. If a spectacularly large, grotesquely twisted nose is successfully reduced to movie-star size, but is crisscrossed with disfiguring scars, the surgeon and the patient both have wasted their time.

Ideally, plastic surgery would leave no scars at all. That is not yet possible. At best, plastic surgery leaves no easily visible scars. Sometimes, even that goal is elusive.

One ineluctable fact of life is that any penetration of the full thickness of the skin will leave a scar. Whether the wound is made with an ax or a scalpel, a scar will result. To deal with this difficult fact, plastic surgeons have adopted two strategies.

The first strategy is to minimize the scar. The second is to hide it.

To minimize scars left by surgery, plastic surgeons use the smallest possible instruments and the most refined tissue-handling techniques. When clamps are needed to close a blood vessel, the plastic surgeon tries to clamp only the bleeding vessel, not the tissue around it. When he cauterizes a blood vessel, he burns only the vessel, avoiding the surrounding tissue. If a large incision is convenient but a small one will do, he goes with the small one. Eliminating unnecessary tissue damage will reduce potential problems with healing, and therefore with scarring.

One of the most common causes of bad scarring is tension across the wound. The tension can be produced in a number of ways. Fluid—loose blood, for example—can collect in the tissue beneath the wound, causing swelling. The swelling, in turn, puts stress on the closed wound by stretching taut the skin around it. Where swelling is a serious threat, drains may be used to relieve fluid pressure. (They are often used in facelifts, draining the incisions behind the ears.)

Normal body or muscle movements may also put stress on a wound. Given a choice in scar placement, a plastic surgeon will put it where there is the least natural tension. Patients are sometimes asked to avoid certain body movements, like stooping, until healing is well under way.

Sutures also create stress. When sewing up a wound, the surgeon tries to put the heaviest binding tension on underlying structures, rather than on the skin surface.

The sutures themselves are kept as small as possible. Thick suture material may leave white "dot" scars where the thread penetrates the skin, even if the incision heals cleanly. Suture material can damage the skin and leave scars in other ways. If the suture material binds too tightly on the surface of the skin, it may leave behind a cross-hatched pattern of dead skin, rather as if the patient had fallen asleep on a tennis racket. The problem is especially serious in areas of heavy sebaceous (oil) gland activity, like the face. And, of course, patients with particularly heavy sebaceous gland activity, like those who suffer from acne problems, are especially at risk.

One option sometimes chosen by plastic surgeons is to use internal sutures. Although not as strong as typical looping stitches, they are sometimes used on patients who have very active skin problems. The actual line of the incision is closed with skin tapes. Healing complications—which can leave a larger incision scar—are somewhat more common with this type of wound closure, but may be a good risk compared to problems posed by conventional looping sutures over sensitive skin.

Even with the best mechanical techniques, it is possible to do further damage to wounds with improper postoperative care. Antiseptics, intended to kill bacteria in a wound, may damage the tissue it was intended to protect. Rather than use harsh antiseptics, most surgeons simply rinse a wound with saline solution until it is clean, and then cover it with a sterile bandage. When a clean wound is closed, the body is usually effective in fighting any germs left behind. In penetrating wounds, like nail wounds, which can't be completely cleaned and closed, antibiotics may be necessary.

If a plastic surgeon uses the smallest instruments, the best techniques, and the best postoperative care, he will still leave a scar anytime he penetrates the full thickness of the skin. It will be a small scar, perhaps no more noticeable than a strand of spiderwebbing, but a scar nevertheless.

So, in addition to minimizing a scar, a good surgeon will also try to hide it.

In ordinary rhinoplasties, the work does leave scars, but only inside the nose where they are not visible. The limited amount of work occasionally done outside the nose is hidden in the folds around the base of the nose. In breast enhancements, the scar is placed in the inframammary fold, where the new, larger breast will fold down. The scar is there and visible, but the breast must be lifted to see it. In breast reductions and reshapings, some scars are hidden behind the breast, some are camouflaged by placing them where the areola blends into the breast skin, and some are simply visible on the face of the breast. The scars on the face of the breast cannot be hidden, so are the subject of the finest, most delicate techniques. Eventually, they will fade to light hairlines.

In eyelid surgery, which removes the loose skin from the lids, the scar is placed precisely within the wrinkle at the top of the lid. The scar can be seen with close inspection, but appears to be an entirely natural facial feature. In tummy tucks, where a visible scar is inevitable, the surgeon still tries to hide it. With clothing. "We put it below the bikini line," Cunningham said.

Some facelift scars—those in front of the ears—cannot be hidden, but by hiding some scars, the surgeons can minimize others. With facelifts, the basic tension-bearing sutures are placed in the hairline, where the scars won't be seen. The sutures on the open face are done with the most delicate stitching, and the scars are practically invisible. And there are always fashionable hairstyles that will obscure them further.

One other complication in scar management primarily involves dark-complected patients and blacks. For reasons not completely understood, dark-complected people are more likely than fair-complected people to develop *keloids*, which are scars that continue to grow and develop longer than normal. The scar tissue may eventually form an unsightly knot, which may itself become an object of aesthetic surgery. Further keloids may or may not follow that second operation.

"Keloids are rare in whites, and not really that common in blacks, but I would hesitate to do purely elective surgery on somebody who had a history of developing keloids. You could wind up with a worse problem than you started with," Cunningham said.

Surgical patients are all individuals, of course, and heal in their own individual patterns. Body chemistry, personal habits, and environment may all affect the way a wound heals and the size of the resulting scar. In all but a very small number of cases, however, well-managed healing will produce a predictable scar.

Tummy Tuck

WITH THE exception of suction lipectomies—the removal of diet-resistant fat pockets from hips, thighs, and buttocks—the most common aesthetic surgeries done below the breasts are tummy tucks. Tummy tucks, which plastic-surgery organizations call abdominoplasties, tighten loose tummy skin and may do other incidental repairs.

One woman said her tummy tuck was done to recover a sense of being attractive, which she had always taken for granted.

"I always thought I was, you know, okay-looking," she said, flashing a quick grin. "Actually, I thought I was good-looking. Then I got pregnant."

A small, pretty, tight-muscled, athletic woman, she gained fifty pounds during the pregnancy, "all of it in front. From the back, you couldn't tell I was pregnant. From the front, I looked like Moby Dick."

After the pregnancy, she worked hard to get rid of the excess weight with diets and exercise. "I even took karate lessons. I tried running for a while, but I think you need a serious mental disease to keep running very long. . . . I mean, it is *intensely* boring."

She lost weight, but found herself with a double handful of

loose skin in the lower abdomen. When exercise didn't seem to tighten it, she went back to her doctor who said, no, in fact, exercise wouldn't do much good. She'd have to live with it.

"It was like, 'So what, you're married. You don't have to be attractive anymore.' "

Then she got unmarried, and the loose skin became something of a preoccupation.

"I was pretty unhappy about it. After the divorce I'd started going out again. Because of my job [in a popular bar near a university] I dated a lot of younger men, and you could see them thinking, Oh, boy, an older woman and she runs a bar. Everything would be fine and then they'd get my clothes off and 'Whoa, what's this?' A couple of them came right out and told me that all that loose skin was a real turnoff."

As part of her follow-up care for an unrelated operation by another surgeon, she was referred to Cunningham. After the examination—the earlier work was fine—Cunningham asked why she hadn't done anything about the loose stomach skin.

"I asked him what he could do. He told me, and I said, 'Terrific, let's do it.' "

Tummy tucks remove unsightly skin on the stomach, but they also leave scars. Because the scars are under stretching pressure, they tend to spread somewhat, sometimes becoming as wide as a pencil.

"The scar never bothered anybody who saw it, not like the loose skin. One guy said something like, what was this, and I said, 'I had a tummy tuck,' and he said, 'Oh, yeah?' and that was the last I heard of it. I've never felt self-conscious about it, and I don't have to worry about wearing a two-piece bathing suit. I think there are a lot of women out there who have a baby or two, and their stomachs get stretched out, and they just don't think they can do anything about it. Well, they can, they ought to. It really does make you look a lot better, and you feel better about yourself," she said.

Is it worth going through a good deal of pain, at substantial expense, to look good for others?

"You hear people say it's weird to worry about your looks, but they're never the people who have problems. I figure if you want to go hang around the swimming pool with your girlfriends, but you're embarrassed to do it, or you're always covering up, or you wear those ugly bathing suits with skirts or something, well, you've got a problem and it's hurting you. You are worrying about it, even if you pretend you aren't. Better to get it fixed."

One of Cunningham's patients (much less the free spirit than the woman interviewed above) decided to seek a tummy tuck after several pregnancies left her with excessive loose skin on her abdomen. A strenuous exercise regime failed to eliminate it.

She also had a clearly visible hernia, or sunken spot, between the two large vertical muscles that covered her abdomen. The hernia was the result of a cesarean section. The tissue joining the two muscles failed to grow back together after they were separated. It's a common problem, relatively minor, and she wanted it repaired.

Cunningham, dressed in light green surgical scrubs, entered the operating room to find the patient sitting on an operating table in a hospital gown, with five other people ready to begin work—an anesthesiologist, a nurse-anesthetist, a surgical tech, and two circulating nurses.

"Okay, now for one of the most embarrassing moments in your entire life, when you get to take off your clothes in front of a bunch of strangers," Cunningham said to the patient. He helped her take off the gown and asked her to stand on a small bench while he sat in front of her and drew freehand a series of ovals within ovals on her abdomen. They were contour lines, he explained, delineating the biggest problem areas.

"When you wear a bikini, would it come down this low, do you think?" Cunningham asked, drawing a long swooping line from the point of one hipbone to the other.

"I don't wear them at all," the patient said.

"We want to make sure that the scar won't be visible whatever you wear," Cunningham said.

The drawing was carefully calculated and took five minutes.

When he finished marking the patient, Cunningham backed away from the table.

"We're going to wash you with a special soap," he told the woman. "We want you to hold your arms away from your sides so you won't contaminate the washed area." A nurse did the washing with a pink antiseptic soap, carefully going over every inch of the woman's trunk.

As the woman was washed, the other members of the operating team were setting up the room. The routine work seemed to relax the patient, who was unavoidably caught in the nerve-racking position of standing nude and motionless while other people handled her, inspected her, and worked around her.

When asked about the sexual implications of medical nudity, Cunningham allows that he knows a pretty woman when he sees one, but is so focused on the job that the sexual element does not intrude. It's a position that doctors always take joshing about, but if you spend any time in an operating room, it becomes obvious that it's the truth. Doctors and nurses see a lot of naked people of every shape, age, and color, and other things are more important than another naked person.

And during an operation, there is something pathetic and un-attractive about a sedated or anesthetized patient. They are so totally helpless, so limp and uncontrolled, that sexual impulses in an observer would seem unnatural.

None of that, naturally, occurs to the patient. So the woman stood nude and nervous until the washing was completed. When it was done, the nurse patted her dry and helped her onto the operating table. The table wings were pulled out to support her arms.

Cunningham had been fighting a badly damaged radio while the woman was washed, and having failed with the tuning dial, began to whack it with his hand.

"Won't do any good," a nurse said. "Somebody dropped it."

Cunningham gave up and tuned in the clearest signal, which happened to be from a pop-rock station, and turned down the volume until it was barely audible. The anesthesiologist had placed an IV needle in the patient's arm and now began feeding her an intravenous anesthetic.

"You should be feeling a little sleepy now," she said, and the woman replied, "A little bit."

Cunningham stepped over and looked down at her and said, "See you in a while." The woman smiled and then suddenly her face went slack as the anesthesia hit.

When she was asleep, Cunningham and the nurse pulled sock-like garments over her legs to help keep her warm during the operation, and then wrapped her legs in elastic bandages.

"One of the dangers of an operation like this is the possibility of thrombosis [blood clot] in the legs and having it extend to the lungs," Cunningham said. "This [wrapping the legs] helps avoid it. It's not a big risk, but there's no point in taking it if you don't have to."

When the patient's legs were wrapped, Cunningham left the operating room to scrub and the nurses bustled around finishing the setup. As they were working, the anesthesiologist indicated one of the woman's breasts and said to a nurse, "Did you notice that auxiliary [extra] nipple there?"

"Yeah, I'm surprised we're not taking that off," the nurse said.

"It's very well developed," the anesthesiologist said. "You don't see one that developed very often."

"What are you talking about?" Cunningham asked as he bumped hip-first into the room, his hands in the air.

"She's got an auxiliary nipple," said the anesthesiologist.

"I'm surprised we're not taking it off," said the nurse.

"Some people like them. There are nerve endings there, and they don't want them off," Cunningham said.

"I'd take it off first thing," the nurse said.

"Some people like them," Cunningham said, with a little iron in his voice.

"I'd still take it off," the nurse said, just as firmly.

Surgical teams often talk in a desultory way about the patients they work upon. The talk is impersonal, if not quite professional—experienced operating-room people have seen virtually every variation on the human body, and every variation of everything that can be done to a body.

Cunningham chats with the others, but will occasionally cut the talk off, especially if it becomes uncomplimentary to the patient.

"I don't care what somebody's personal opinions are about a patient, if they think the patient is vain or stupid or whatever. It is their responsibility to take care of that person to the best of their ability. When somebody makes a [denigrating] comment, it indicates that their personal opinions could be intruding on their professional responsibilities, and they need to be reminded what they think about the patient doesn't matter. If they can't do their best, get out. And you know, I do find it a little bit annoying to hear rude comments about somebody who is lying there unconscious and can't defend herself."

Like breast reductions, a tummy tuck can be a bloody business. The operation is conceptually straightforward: the abdominal skin is tightened by taking out a large band of skin and fat just below the navel, and the top and bottom edges of the cut are sewn together.

In addition to the normal problems of serious surgery, such as control of blood loss, a major aesthetic problem of a tummy tuck is making the two edges of the wound heal neatly. The layers of skin and fat at the navel level are usually thicker than the layers of skin and fat across the pelvis. Since these two areas will be joined, some lipectomy—fat removal—is needed to even out the two layers of flesh. If it's not done, there will be a ledge, or bump, along the suture line.

Cunningham began the operation with a long, curving incision that ran from one point of the pelvis to the other, swooping down over the pubic area. The line would more or less parallel the top edge of a pair of bikini underpants, but slightly lower. The incision went in deep—nearly an inch—before completely penetrating the layer of fat below the skin.

"That's not much fat," Cunningham commented. "She's really in pretty good shape."

(The amount of fat on people ostensibly in good condition can shock first-time surgical observers. The fat layer routinely runs an inch or two thick even on people not obviously overweight.)

With the initial incision made, Cunningham began removing fat from the abdominal area, using the technique called suction lipectomy. While most plastic surgery is notable for its cool finesse, a lipectomy is brutal work. It is done, essentially, with a vacuum cleaner and a steel tube as a pickup. The tube has suction holes on one end and what looks like a bicycle grip on the other, with the vacuum cleaner hose running out behind the bicycle grip.

To remove fat, the surgeon makes an incision and then pushes—rams—the tube through the fat cells, literally tearing them apart. The vacuum sucks fat, fluid, and blood out of the resulting cavity. The surgeon has to push hard to break through the fat cells but, at the same time, carefully avoid damage to the overlying or underlying tissue.

Cunningham thrust the vacuum pickup, called a cannula, under the skin dozens of times, removing a half-liter of fat and fluid.

"Okay, now that should feather down pretty well," he said, indicating the belly skin. "When we cut off the bottom strip it should fit right in [to the incision along the panty line]."

With the lipectomy finished, he put the cannula aside and used a scalpel and cautery to begin separating abdominal skin and fat from the underlying muscle.

"I'd like to go up as far as the ribs, but I don't think we'll be able to, with this scar here," he said, touching a scar just below the woman's rib cage. It had been left by an earlier gallbladder operation.

The work was slow, as it usually is, Cunningham working five or six inches under the layer of belly skin. When he had undermined as much abdominal skin as possible, he located the hernia and quickly sewed the two separated muscles together. The suture material looked like thick, tough, fish line. The hernia would never actually heal, so the sutures must hold for the rest of the woman's life.

"Leaving the sutures is no problem," Cunningham explained. "The stuff is nonreactive with the body."

Asked if it would hold for forty or fifty years, he said, "Listen, if they open her coffin a thousand years from now, they're going to find a bunch of dust and a piece of perfectly good fish line."

The hernia sewed up neatly, with Cunningham working freely under the woman's abdominal skin, as though it were a loose T-shirt.

When he finished with the hernia, the woman was left with loose skin between the panty-line incision and her rib cage, except where the skin was tacked to underlying muscle by her navel. Cunningham picked up a scalpel and made a vertical incision from the center of the horizontal panty-line cut upward to the navel, and then cut around the navel. Isolated from its supporting skin, the navel stuck out of the wound like a tiny Three Mile Island cooling tower.

The skin had now been loosened over the entire abdomen. Cunningham asked that the woman be flexed into a semi-seated position. That position would cause the abdomen to collapse inward and allow the skin to be drawn tighter without putting too much strain on the stitches. As she was being flexed forward, her body suddenly spasmed.

"She didn't like that," Cunningham said, looking sharply at the anesthesiologist.

"It was the airway," the anesthesiologist said, sounding abashed. "She's deep enough for the surgery but not deep enough for the [airway] tube."

As the level of anesthesia was increased slightly, Cunningham explained: "She was coughing. Evolution has given us a pretty violent reaction to anything in the airway. If you can't protect your airway with a cough or a gag, you're in trouble."

When she was ready to be moved again, the circulating nurses and the anesthesiologist helped push the patient to a flexed position. When her body was comfortably solid, Cunningham pulled the loose abdominal skin down over her pelvic area and tacked it in place with several quick stitches. The stretching elongated

107

the navel opening and pulled it right down to the panty-line incision, giving her abdominal skin the look of a T-shirt with a hole.

The tightness of the skin is purely a matter of judgment. If it's stretched too much, pressure on the incision line can cause problems with healing, and later create a larger-than-necessary scar. On the other hand, if it's not tight enough, the basic objective of the operation has failed and the woman is left with both extra abdominal skin and a tummy-tuck scar.

(In a completely different tummy-tuck operation, Cunningham tacked the skin in place and asked, mostly rhetorically, "That tight enough?"

"Looks tight to me," said the resident who was assisting with the operation. And a minute later: "You know anything about her?"

"I know she gives piano lessons," Cunningham said.

"With a nice tight tummy like that she'll be sitting up straight at the keyboard. Because she *can't* lean back," the resident said. The nurse and the anesthesiologist laughed and Cunningham wiggled his eyebrows and said, "Jeez, you could probably get a paper out of that."

But the joking apparently worried him a bit, because he pressed the skin along the line and farther up the stomach, peering down over his mask before he shook his head: "Nah, it's fine. It's just right.")

With the skin temporarily tacked in place, there remained a band of fat and skin hanging over the pelvis below the sutures. Cunningham quickly sliced it away.

To begin the closing of the panty-line incision, Cunningham anchored the top of the cut to the bottom with several heavy individual stitches placed a couple of inches apart.

With the wound's edges lined up and anchored, Cunningham made a quick crisscross where the navel could be seen tenting the skin, pulled the navel through, and sewed it in place.

"Some people just do a vertical slit and leave it at that. I find you get too much pressure on it that way and wind up with a belly button that's almost invisible," Cunningham said. "I like to make a star-shaped incision. You get a better look that way."

In this case, he was dissatisfied with the look, because there was an extra tiny lump of fat on one side of the navel, under the skin. The lump distorted the navel opening, so Cunningham cut loose several stitches, snipped out the extra fat, and restitched the opening.

With the navel in place, he went back to the main panty-line incision and finished closing it, using a long running stitch. As he was working he asked the nurse how much saline solution had been fed into the woman: "That's the second liter, right?" he said, nodding at a plastic bottle on an overhead rack.

"Right. She's got two hundred [cubic centimeters] in her from the second bottle."

"Good. Better that she pees all night than not at all," Cunningham said.

"Are you going to want to sew in those drains?" asked a nurse. Cunningham had earlier mentioned that he planned to insert surgical drains in the wound.

"Yeah, I will."

"What do you want?"

"A couple of ten-millimeter Jackson-Pratts."

The nurse went to get them, and Cunningham explained that the raw surfaces created by the lipectomy would "weep" a large amount of fluid into the wound. The body could absorb it, but there would be much less trauma to surrounding tissue if it were drained away.

When the nurse returned with the drains ("Jackson-Pratt hubless 10mm wide flat silicone drain perforated ¾ length, 20 centimeters long") Cunningham inserted them deep into the wound and stitched them in place. The outside ends of the drain tubes would later be inserted in separate plastic bottles that look a little like old-fashioned "pineapple" hand grenades.

When he was finished sewing, Cunningham stepped back and looked down at the patient. The supine woman looked hurt: there was a long, angry-looking incision across her pelvic area, running from the point of one hip to the other.

"She's going to look fine," Cunningham said as he peeled off his gloves. "The scar will be okay, and her body'll look terrific."

Recovery time on a routine tummy tuck is ten days to two weeks, but that could lengthen if there is skin or soft-tissue loss.

"You can get scarring, you can lose some skin or soft tissue, and the belly button may not survive. Except for the scarring— there's always some of that—those things don't happen very commonly, but they can happen," Cunningham said.

Tummy tucks are growing in popularity with the American public. Plastic surgeons did some 32,340 of them in 1986, up from some 20,900 in 1984. That's a 55 percent increase over two years.

And though they are popular, tummy tucks hurt.

"I felt bad for a while, for a few days. It was a couple of more weeks before I could get around without hurting. It wasn't terrible, but I felt like I didn't want to make any sudden moves, you know?" said the woman who ran the bar.

"How bad was it? I'd do it again, in a minute. It hurt, but I got back to work pretty quick. I think it might lay some people up for a while, and other people, it won't bother them. Like when you get a wisdom tooth pulled. Some people are running around an hour later, and some people stay in bed for three days," she said.

Snapshot: A Priesthood

I was in the emergency room during the evening, watching procedures and interviewing the doctors. At some point, during what began as a slow night, one of the doctors started talking about a common metaphor: the surgeon as latter-day priest.

A little before midnight, a nurse and a medical student sat in the staff lounge and laughed about it. The nurse had ice-blue Scandinavian eyes and natural streaky blond hair and was pretty. The medical student was a smart kid with glasses.

Then a bad case came in. The OR nurses said it was one of the worst they'd seen, in a man still alive.

The patient arrived by helicopter from farm country northwest of the Twin Cities. There were thunderstorms floating around in the warm night sky, and the radio link between St. Paul–Ramsey Medical Center and the chopper wasn't as good as it might have been.

The on-board nursing crew was talking on the radio of burns and tearing injuries and massive doses of morphine. The injuries came out of a tractor accident. The emergency-room doctors speculated that the farmer had been pinned under a hot engine. That happens occasionally, out in farm country, along with other spectacularly cruel and bloody accidents. This one would be different. And worse.

The chopper landed a couple of hundred feet from the emergency room entrance. The patient was manhandled out of the chopper onto a hospital gurney; bottles of saline solution hung on an overhead rack. He was taken to an evaluation room, where the doctors stood and looked and shook their heads, then he was shipped upstairs to Room 10, the emergency operating room.

The patient was a young man. He had been plowing when the

tractor rolled on him, trapping him beneath one of the huge wheels. The tractor was in gear, and the wheel kept going round and round, chewing into his left hip, leg, and back with its massive tread. The wound looked precisely like a tractor-tire track in a muddy black-dirt field.

The very grinding action that cut into the man's body helped keep him alive: the friction was so great that the wheel burned his flesh as it cut through his body, cauterizing the wound and reducing the loss of blood. The flesh that wasn't torn free was charred black.

A nine-member trauma team tried to salvage what was left. They included a general surgeon and two residents, an anesthesiologist, a nurse-anesthetist, two circulating nurses, an X-ray technician and a surgical tech. They worked fast, but without panic, to get the operation going.

Once on the table, the farmer was quickly and efficiently catheterized. A white plastic tube was pushed up his penis to the bladder, and a special dye pumped inside. Then X rays were taken. If the bladder showed on the X ray as a sharply defined circle, it was probably intact. If the X ray showed dye feathering from the bladder into the abdominal cavity, it was probably damaged. That would be more big trouble.

The lead surgeon also did a peritoneal lavage, which involves pumping a solution into the abdominal cavity and then sucking it out again with a large needle. The fluid is examined for blood cells, and if any are found, the patient is assumed to be suffering internal bleeding.

As the tests were made, the anesthesiologist was setting up for the operation: taping the patient's eyes shut, inserting new IV needles in his arm. A breathing tube was placed deep in his throat. (Candidates for routinely scheduled surgery are told not to eat beforehand. In trauma cases, where times and types of food intake are not known, special procedures are needed to guard against the possibility that the patient might vomit and choke on his own vomit.)

As the preliminaries continued, the lead surgeon finished his own examination and stepped into the hallway, shaking his head, his face grim.

"The left leg is gone," he said. "It's dead. The right leg is alive, but we don't know if we can keep it alive. He has a major defect on his right side, on the back, the hip, and the leg, and one testicle is crushed—I've got urology coming up to take it off. If we saved the right leg, I don't know how much function he'd have left. I've got an orthopedist coming up to take a look at it. Even if the muscles are okay, the main nerve there, the sciatic nerve, is so close to the burned area that it might have been cooked. We have to look at that. He's also got air down there in the [right] leg. We see that in this kind of accident. It gets pumped down there. If there's any debris, any rubber or grease, the leg is gone."

The good news was that there was no apparent internal bleeding, and the patient's bladder was intact. The orthopedic surgeon arrived, and he and the general surgeon conferred over the patient's legs. They decided to remove the left one immediately, and to try to clean up the right leg so that it could be watched for a couple of days.

As they were talking, the speakers in the hallway ceiling came alive: "Surgery stat Room Ten. Surgery stat Room Ten."

"There goes the night, " said one of the nurses. "Room 10" is the hospital's general term for the emergency operating suites. In this case, the actual Room 10 was already occupied, so they ran into Room 9, next to the operating room where the farmer was, and began getting it ready for immediate surgery.

The lead surgeon, who had been with the farmer, walked out and said, "What's up?"

"There's a stab wound in the chest on the way up," a nurse said.

A few seconds later, the emergency-room people rolled another surgical cart through the door, this one carrying a young man who was lying flat on his back. He had been stabbed near the left nipple, in the lower abdomen and the right back. He was fully conscious, but smelled of alcohol. He was taken into Room 9, and as he was prepped the chief surgical resident began questioning him.

"You're a pretty healthy fellow, huh? You been drinking? You take any street drugs? How old are you? Did anybody hit you on the head? You ever have any lung problems? Diabetes? Kidney problems?"

"No, no, no . . ."

"Sir," the chief resident told the man, "you have a potentially life-threatening injury and we want to operate to see if you're bleeding inside. You have a stab wound in the back right over where your liver is."

"I feel fine."

"If it got your liver, you won't feel fine in the morning, let me clue you."

For the next two hours, the lead surgeon shuttled between the two operating rooms, overseeing both operations at the same time. The orthopedic surgeon took off the farmer's leg, and it was bundled off down the hall in a plastic bag by one of the nurses. The chief surgical resident opened up the stab victim, checked his liver, and began checking his intestines for cuts that might pump waste matter into his intestinal cavity.

Eventually, the stab victim was wheeled down the dark hallways to the recovery room, and two hours later, the farmer followed.

When they were gone, the doctors stood in the hall outside the OR talking about the night and shaking their masked heads.

The streaky-haired nurse peeled off her mask and threw it in a waste receptacle and walked wearily back to the lounge for a cup of coffee. Her hair had gone flyaway and she no longer looked so pretty. The farmer, she said, was a particularly depressing case because he was so young and in such good physical health. A decent, hardworking man who normally would have had decades of life ahead of him, unlike some of the scumbags brought in here. Now, she thought, the farmer would die if he was lucky. (He made it out of the recovery room, only to die two days later in the intensive-care unit. The cause of death was heart failure.)

And it was a good thing, said the nurse, that there weren't television cameras in Room 10. If the public could see a radical emergency surgery, like the one done on the farmer, they might stop treating surgeons like priests; nothing holy happened in the surgery that night. It was more like butchery, and damn rough work, too. The surgeons cut and pumped blood and sewed and hoped and still shook their heads. All their skill made little difference. Maybe the only thing that would make a difference was prayer.

"Were you here the night when they brought in that quad?" she asked. Yeah. "You feel so bad. The guy doesn't even hurt, and he's got nothing left. Nothing anybody can do about it. You feel so bad."

It was another common-enough summertime story.

A young man dove off a boat without checking the water depth and hit his head on the bottom of the river. The impact displaced a vertebra, crushing his spinal cord. He was rushed to the medical center, feeling no pain at all. Nor would he ever again feel pain below the neck. The chief orthopedic surgeon came in, wearing weekend jeans and sneakers, and the radiologist handed him some X rays, and he pinned one up on a light window, studied it for a few seconds, and said, "Shit."

Outside in the hallway, the young girlfriend, the seat of her jeans still wet from water leaking through from her bathing suit, was drinking a cup of machine coffee and chatting animatedly with a nurse. A few minutes later a gray-faced couple came through, and she walked up to them and said the guy was in the examining room and she thought he'd be okay.

These were the kid's parents. It would be a couple of hours before they found that their son was now a quadriplegic.

"It always happens to the athletes, because it's always the lively guys who jump in head first without looking," the streaky-haired nurse said dispiritedly.

"They could look at that [X-ray] film and tell that he was gone. Praying is about the only thing he's got. It's about the only thing he can do," she said.

So the nurse was not in a mood to grant surgeons their priestly status. The night had been too rough, and there was still the stink of blood and cooked flesh in her hair. And when miracles had been needed, all the surgeons could deliver was skill and knowledge.

Still, the similarities between surgeons and Old Testament priests are numerous. Surgeons have the prestige, the wealth, the exclusive knowledge, and even the guild status once given only to a priesthood.

And the ritual is similar.

Surgeons begin their careers as novices. They are inducted into mysteries too arcane for the commonality during a passage of terror and intense stress, called medical school. After the novitiate, they enter a period of apprenticeship, assisting the full-fledged surgeons in their duties.

These duties are performed wearing special garments, in obsessively clean and secret rooms buried within enormous, expensive temples of medicine. All of it—the procedure, the paraphernalia—is kept well away from the prying eyes of the masses and, usually, away even from the eyes of the patient, who is rendered unconscious with any of a variety of special potions and gases.

The surgeon does the critical work, the cutting, surrounded by a group of acolytes, also specially robed, who assist him, and even speak in strange tongues—"anterior," they say, when they mean "front."

Conclusive certification of a surgeon's status as a priest comes later, but not too much later: the bill. Nothing about a really good priesthood comes cheap, whether the payment is made in bullocks, gold bangles, or dollar bills.

Like all priesthoods, surgeons have their secrets. Failure is not one of them. All priesthoods must learn to deal with failure, surgeons no less than any other. Sometimes, things just don't work. The doctors never had a chance with the farmer. They never had a chance with the kid who broke his neck. Everybody knows it, and no blame attaches.

But there are secrets. Surgeons sometimes rant and rave and throw their tools. They make unkind comments about their patients and about other doctors and about the hospitals they work in. They sometimes do stupid things.

The argument that doctors make up a latter-day priesthood can be pushed too far, of course. The game, after a while, grows tiresome, and objections begin to crop up.

But before the analogy is abandoned, consider a final story.

Cunningham and two other men, all dressed in the blue surgical scrub suits and paper booties worn in surgery, walked down to the hospital's public cafeteria. The cafeteria was crowded with the lunch-hour rush. They paid for their meals and waited a moment until a table cleared out at the edge of the room.

When they sat down, Cunningham started talking about the topography of a facelift just completed, until one of the others leaned forward and said quietly, "You can feel the people looking at us. It's like a physical wave of approval."

Cunningham grinned and said, "Yeah."

Later, when the afternoon's work was done, Cunningham stood in the hospital locker room and peeled off his scrub suit, balled it up, and fired it at a half-filled laundry basket.

"You know that feeling of approval you were talking about?" he asked. "You get hooked on it. A lot of surgeons sneak scrubs out of the hospital and wear them around the house. They like to feel like surgeons, and they like people to see them in scrubs. They like that approval. You really get hooked."

Surgeons *like* being priests. It feels *terrific*. It feels absolutely *wonderful*.

Suction Lipectomy

The woman took off her robe for the preop exam and stepped toward the table where she would sit. From the back, her problem was evident: she was slender enough, but the outside edge of her upper thighs flared out, as though she were wearing jodhpurs.

THE BIGGEST aesthetic problem of the American middle class can be summed in a single unhappy word: fat. And, for the most part, plastic and reconstructive surgeons can't do much about it.

"Everybody's heard about suction lipectomies, but they're not for fat people. The best candidates for lipectomies are people who are in pretty good shape," said Cunningham.

A suction lipectomy removes deposits of body fat by physically piercing and crushing fat cells. The surgical debris is sucked out with an instrument that is essentially a vacuum cleaner.

Suction lipectomies are the most popular aesthetic surgeries done today. According to statistics compiled by the American Society of Plastic and Reconstructive Surgeons, some 99,330 suction lipectomies were done in 1986, up 78 percent over 1984, when there were 55,900 cases.

That statistic is particularly amazing since the operation was only developed (in Europe) in the mid-1970s, and was barely known in America until the 1980s.

Most suction lipectomies are done on the thighs, abdomen, and buttocks. Some are done on the face and neck, and a few in other locations, depending upon the individual patient and his or her particular problem.

"The best candidates, the typical candidates, are the people who work out, and who have good bodies, but they've got these pockets of diet-resistant fat that won't go away. We can go in and get the fat for them," Cunningham said. Typical examples are "saddlebags" on women's hips and "love handles" on men. One of Cunningham's clients ran a workout studio and found the pouches of fat on her hips and on her thighs below the buttocks were unacceptable for business reasons.

"I guess it made her clients wonder exactly how much good the workouts would do them, if she [the instructor] still had the bulges," Cunningham said.

Why not take fat off grossly obese people with suction lipectomies? There are several good reasons. Here are three.

First, the skin on fat people has often been severely and permanently stretched out of shape—the same problem women face with skin that won't tighten up after a pregnancy. With obese people, however, the problem is global, rather than confined to the lower abdomen.

"If you just sucked all the fat out, the skin would fit the person like a loose sock or a loose shirt. He'd have a bigger aesthetic problem with the skin than he did with the fat, and you couldn't get it to tighten up evenly no matter what you did," Cunningham said.

A second reason for not using suction to remove large amounts of body fat is that the technique destroys the blood vessels that run from the layers of muscle through the layers of fat to the skin. If you destroy too much fat, along with the penetrating blood vessels, the overlying skin will die. That does not happen with local suction lipectomies because neighboring blood vessels can compensate for those destroyed.

If a substantial area of skin dies, the patient is in serious trouble, just as if he had suffered a serious burn. The only medical techniques for handling the problem involve skin grafts, which often leave disfiguring scars.

A third reason for not using suction to remove large amounts of body fat is that the body could not tolerate it.

"The trauma [of a suction lipectomy] creates an outflow of fluids from the body, just like it would on a burn," Cunningham said. "On a burn, though, the fluid weeps out of the surface of the skin. A suction lipectomy is like an internal burn, and the fluid weeps out of the raw surfaces of the fat and into the wound. To replace that, these patients need a massive amount of fluid. If we suck out 500 cc (a little more than a pint) of blood and fatty fluid, we feel that they should get three times that, or about 1,500 cc of replacement fluid. If we take out 1,200 to 1,500 cc, we feel they'll need a transfusion."

The removal of 1,500 cc, or about a quart and a half of fluid, is not much in terms of a really obese person, but it is considered a serious surgical matter, Cunningham said. To simply suck out fifty pounds of fat would create an uncontrollable and probably fatal wound.

One typical suction lipectomy began on a warm summer morning at University Hospitals, on a small, athletic patient who had already had a tummy tuck. Now she wanted pockets of fat removed from her hips, thighs, and abdomen.

Cunningham had her disrobe and spent several minutes drawing on the areas where she needed work. She was no stranger to the operating room: in addition to the tummy tuck, she had had a subcutaneous mastectomy some years before, after a precancerous condition was detected. In a subcutaneous mastectomy, only the fat and gland of the breast are removed, and the skin is left. After that operation, her breasts had been rebuilt with silicone implants.

As Cunningham drew on her, a nurse-anesthetist came into the room and said, "Hi, I'm Bill, the nurse-anesthetist."

"Are you going to give me something that won't make me throw up?" the woman asked.

"Have you thrown up after anesthesia before?" Bill asked.

"I sure did last time, boy," she said.

"Well, we'll have to give you the special stuff this time," the nurse-anesthetist said. He left to find the special stuff.

Cunningham was still drawing on her body, and without looking up, asked, "You bring the girdle?"

"Right over your head," she said. She reached over him, into a cabinet, and pulled out a thick old-fashioned girdle. "It's my mother's, it's not a Sears," she said.

"That's okay. We only tell people to get a Sears because they work okay, but this is fine," Cunningham said.

"It's pretty tight, you're going to have to grease me up to get me in there," she said.

"We'll get a couple of people jammers," said a medical student, who had come into the room behind Cunningham. "You know, like the ones they have on the Japanese subways, smash you right in there."

Cunningham finished his drawing and helped the woman into a blue robe and asked her to sit on the operating table so the nurse-anesthetist, who had come back into the room, could insert the IV.

"You're going to feel a little Minnesota mosquito bite now," said the nurse-anesthetist. He gave her a small shot of novocaine, waited until the skin was numb, and put in the IV needle.

"You haven't had anything to eat since midnight?" asked the nurse-anesthetist.

"No, and since before that, too. I haven't even had a drink of water."

"Good. Good."

When the nurse-anesthetist was finished, Cunningham asked the patient to hop off the table again, cross her hands over her chest, and grab her opposite shoulders, so a nurse could scrub her. The scrubbed area would extend from her breasts to just below her knees.

"Now [the patient] here is thirty-three, which is fine, but you don't want to get into this operation too much past the mid-forties. The skin starts losing its flexibility and that can cause some problems during recovery," Cunningham said.

"Am I going to be as swollen as I was when I got the tummy tuck?" the woman asked.

"Not so severely, no."

"So I'll be able to wear regular clothes?"

"Well, maybe you'll want to go with peasant styles for a while, something loose. . . ."

When the scrubbing was finished, the nurses began to blot the patient dry with sterile towels, using a good stack of towels before they finished. "Surgery's cheap, you know," Cunningham muttered. "It's all these sheets we use up, that's what costs . . ."

When the patient was dry, she lay back across the table, and her legs were covered with drapes. An anesthesiologist came in, checked the anesthesia setup, talked a couple of minutes with the nurse-anesthetist, and started the anesthesia.

"We'll try something a little different this time," the anesthesiologist said. "I think you'll like it better."

"Is this the stuff that tastes like garlic?" asked Cunningham.

"Yeah, coming right up."

"I can feel it," said the patient, continuing her nonchalant attitude.

"She runs a world-class restaurant, I hope it's the better garlic," Cunningham said.

"See you later, guys," the patient said and went to sleep.

Cunningham went out to scrub as the anesthesiologist continued hooking up his monitoring equipment.

"She's a nice-looking little lady," he said as he worked.

"Yeah, but look at the scars," said a nurse. "What, she's had a breast enhancement and tummy tuck, and now this?"

Cunningham came back a few moments later, hands in the air, and the surgical tech hustled around to get his gown and gloves.

"What's she trying to do, make herself into the perfect woman?" said the nurse who had commented on the scars.

"I think she's just trying to look her best," Cunningham said with a drop-dead tone.

"But the deformity certainly isn't gross," said the medical student.

"No, but the aesthetics are really in the eye of the beholder, aren't they?" asked Cunningham.

Another nurse asked, "What's she had done? Did she have an augmentation?"

"No, she had a sub-cu mastectomy by Dr. ———. Looks pretty good, huh?"

"Yeah, it does."

"And she had that tummy tuck about nine months ago," Cunningham said.

Before beginning the operation, Cunningham and the surgical tech covered most of the patient's body with sterile blankets and rolled long white cotton tubes up her legs to keep them warm. When they were finished, only the operating field, the abdomen, was still exposed. Two medical students came into the room with their scrubbed hands in the air, but Cunningham, the surgical tech, and the circulating nurse ignored them until the patient was covered. Then the surgical tech and circulator helped them robe and glove.

While they were doing that, Cunningham, using a long, flexible needle, made two dozen injections of a local anesthetic to the thighs, hips, and legs. The anesthetic, lidocaine, also contained epinephrine to constrict the blood vessels and limit blood loss.

"Fat tissue contains a good rich blood supply so you want to get as much constriction as possible," Cunningham said.

When he was finished injecting, he waited a moment, then picked up a scalpel and made two short incisions at the points of the pelvis. Neither was more than two inches long. From there, he could work the entire stomach area, and well down into the hips and legs, with no further cutting.

The actual lipectomy procedure is accomplished with a tool called a cannula, which looks like a short stainless-steel curtain rod. One end is blunt and rounded, with a hole on the bottom side. At the other end, where the surgeon holds it, is a molded plastic grip that looks like a bicycle handle. A vacuum tube runs out the end of the grip to a vacuum canister on the floor. In other words, the whole apparatus can be accurately described as a vacuum cleaner with a short pickup wand.

Holding the incision open with his fingers, Cunningham pushed the cannula into the stomach area under the skin, piercing and smashing the fat cells that got in the way. The vacuum had not yet been turned on.

"The idea is to pretunnel so you can get a better idea of where you are in the whole process," Cunningham said. The work is physical: he has to ram the rod through the fat. Once it was under, he pumped it back and forth, back and forth, methodically working below the skin of most of the lower abdomen.

When he had pretunneled the stomach areas, he asked the nurse to turn on the vacuum, which the nurse called a "slurp." The machine itself looked a little as though a child tried to make a *Star Wars* R2D2 robot out of a couple of Mason jars and a toy wagon. When it was turned on, a nasty-looking gruel of fat, blood, and serum began flowing into the slurp's transparent plastic receptacle.

"You can control the cannula better if you keep your fingers on the tip. You can get an idea of how deep you're in and what you're getting," Cunningham said to the med student as he worked. "You've got to remember that you're only sucking where the tip is, so you don't have to pump the whole thing in and out."

He was sweating lightly with the effort of working the pickup.

"How badly will she be bruised?"

"She'll be very black and blue wherever we work . . . and she'll form a lot of scar tissue [under the skin], but in this case that's good, because it'll help pull the skin back together," said Cunningham.

Good lipectomies, Cunningham explained, leave a thin layer of fat attached to the skin and concentrate on removing the lower fat layers in the target area. "If you take the fat right off the skin, you can get a dimpling effect. If you leave a thin layer, you can avoid that, and get a smoother contour," he said.

An off-duty nurse came into the operating room and asked if she could watch. She'd had a lipectomy herself a few months earlier, she said, and wanted to see one.

"Did it hurt?" asked the med student.

"Oh, yeah, it hurt quite a bit the first two weeks, and the bruising was terrible, but they all faded out and now there isn't any sign of it. My weight and clothing sizes didn't change at all, you know, but I look better. I don't stick out around my legs; I had these lumps. My sister is coming in for the operation, so it must be genetics that does it to you."

Cunningham stepped down to the foot of the operating table and squinted up at the patient.

"Wouldn't you say she was a little trimmer over here?" he asked the general public, pointing to the left side of the woman's stomach.

"Yes, but she looked a little trimmer there before the operation, too," said the circulating nurse.

"She wanted that evened up," said Cunningham. "We need to take the contour down a little bit." As in so many aesthetic surgeries, Cunningham said, getting everything symmetrical is a big part of the work.

"How much saline are you giving her?" asked the med student.

"We try to shoot for three times as much as the fluid we take out." Cunningham glanced at the vacuum on the floor and its growing accumulation of fluid. "How much have we got out, exactly?"

"About 600 cc's," said the circulating nurse. "We've got the second liter of saline going in."

Because so much fluid is taken out during a suction lipectomy, and so much more weeps into the wound, a lot of fluid must be replaced in the body to maintain blood pressure, Cunningham said.

"If you get low blood pressure, you can get a situation where the patient's heart is pumping along, trying to get blood out everywhere it's needed, but just barely managing. Then she sits up suddenly, gravity pulls a bunch of blood down into the legs, and the heart's unable to pump enough to the brain, and she keels over. If the situation was bad enough, she could have a seizure. You can avoid that by keeping the blood pressure up.

"The other reason for putting in a lot of fluid is that it keeps the kidneys working well. If she gets really dehydrated, she could go into kidney failure. It's better to have her urinating into a catheter than trying to rescue her after a [kidney] failure."

The operation went quickly, as quickly as any that he does. Cunningham finished the abdominal area and then, simply by changing his position, began tunneling the fatty pouches on the patient's buttocks and thighs, still working through the small hip-bone incisions. When he had finished and had done several touch-ups, he withdrew the cannula and quickly sutured the short incisions.

"Now comes the hard part, getting her into that damn girdle," he said. He explained that the girdle was used to hold the skin firmly against the raw face of the underlying tissue to promote quick healing.

It took four people working hard to get the girdle on the patient: she was an awkward bundle, floppy, still attached to the IV and breathing apparatus, and she couldn't be gripped too tightly without bruising her. When the girdle was finally on, Cunningham used a pair of surgical scissors to cut out the crotch so the patient could urinate.

"The girdle will have to stay on for three weeks," he said.

Finished with the patient, Cunningham stripped off the sterile operating robe and gloves and picked up the file of paperwork that accompanies every operation. He filled it out carefully, working on a tool tray and talking with the anesthesiologist about the amounts of drugs used in the procedure. The anesthesiologist was bringing the patient up as they talked.

"Hey, wake up there," he said, peering down at her face. She smiled groggily, and the nurses lifted her off the table and slid her onto a hospital gurney. A little more than an hour after

Cunningham had started drawing on her stomach, she was wheeled out of the operating room to the recovery area.

A few weeks later, talking about her operation, the woman said that she judged it to be worthwhile and declared herself satisfied. It had taken out the bulges that she so despised, although the process had hurt.

"It seemed like I couldn't sit down for a week. God, it hurt. Of all the operations I had, it was probably the most painful. The thing is, you can't go easy on it, if it's your bottom. If you want to walk, sit, bend over, do anything, it's going to hurt," she said.

The bruising was also bad, she said, but didn't bother her so much because nobody could see it, and it faded fairly quickly.

"I look better, but it did hurt," she said.

There are difficulties associated with suction lipectomies.

A few people have died from them, although the number is probably less than a dozen, a good score considering that several hundred thousand have been done by now. Most of those deaths have been associated with surgeons not specifically trained in the procedure.

Suction lipectomies do produce significant soreness and bruising, and for a week or so after the operation, the patient will look much worse than before it was done—it takes a while for the healing processes to work.

On the other hand, Cunningham said, suction lipectomies are the quickest and safest ways to get rid of those unwanted lumps and bumps that afflict even the best-conditioned people.

And they have made obsolete what only a few years ago was a favorite operation, the fanny tuck.

"That tuck looked all right under clothes, but it left serious scarring. You don't get the scarring with the lipectomies, and the result is just as good or better, so bye-bye fanny tucks," Cunningham said.

Snapshot: Ethics

One day in an operating room at St. Paul–Ramsey Medical Center, a senior resident surgeon, a junior resident, a nurse, and a surgical tech were preparing for an operation. Cunningham, who would do the work, had not yet arrived. The senior resident asked the junior if there was blood immediately available in case the patient needed a transfusion.

"Ah, well, a nurse said something about it, so I think they've done that," said the junior. The nurse was not in the operating room at the moment.

"Well, I mean, is it?" asked the senior.

"Well, the nurse . . . I don't know. I don't know if it's ready or not," said the junior.

The senior resident made a note to ask the nurse about the blood. When she returned, she told him that blood was on order and waiting.

That afternoon, the day's operations done, Cunningham sat in a restaurant, drank a glass of wine, and listened to an account of the exchange. The junior's answer, he said, represented one of the more important moments in the young man's brief career.

"When you're learning to be a surgeon, there's this intense pressure always to know. You're always expected to know, and you never want to admit that you don't know. But nobody knows everything, all the time," Cunningham said.

"One of the few inexcusable errors in surgery is to wing it, to fake it when somebody's health is on the line. If you say you know, and you don't know, and that causes an adverse outcome in the case, that's inexcusable.

"We [university surgeons] can be very forgiving of technical errors or errors caused by inexperience. If you're training someone, and he shows that he won't make the same error twice, and shows good judgment based on what he knows, then we can have confidence that he can be trained.

"But if he said he knew the blood was ready, and he didn't know, and it wasn't, that's a normative error. He's guilty of telling a lie that could kill somebody. If the guy's gotten this far, and he doesn't understand right from wrong, then he just doesn't have the right stuff. He's committed the fatal error, an error that can't be corrected."

It's difficult to talk with surgeons about ethics. Their most serious ethical problems are intensely situational: an ethical decision in one case might not be ethical in a virtually identical case. Other ethical problems are invisible. If the junior resident had said confidently, "Yes, the blood is ready," he would have been accurate. No harm would have come to the patient, should she have needed a routine transfusion. He would have maintained his image of knowledgeability. He most likely would convince even himself that he "knew." But, Cunningham would argue, he would nevertheless have a severe ethical problem—he simply wouldn't have been found out. Not even by himself.

There are also ambiguous cases, where behavior may be unethical, but then, may not be.

"Some things are clearly wrong. Phony operations, or those stories you hear about surgeons lighting up a cigarette in the operating room and dripping ashes into the wound—but those things aren't hard calls. Everybody recognizes those. The hard calls are the ethical problems you're not even aware of, if you don't actually think about them and talk about them.

"Some surgeons operate when they don't have to. Say you have a borderline case, and you're not busy, and there are financial pressures from your hospital administrators and partners to stay busy, and bring the money in. So you say, 'What the heck—the guy really needs the work.' If you're not careful, you could find yourself doing work that might be better handled with more conservative treatment. But you see, what you do *worked*. So is it unethical?" Cunningham asked.

Ethics may also involve small decisions—whether to accept a reasonable result as good enough, when you could make it fractionally better by spending more time with it.

"Say you're doing a suction lipectomy and you're pretty much done, and then you start thinking, Well, if I spend another half hour dinking around, I can probably even it out a little more over here. . . .

"You could say, The heck with it, that's good enough, and go play golf. Who's to know? There's nobody else in the operating room who could make the call on something like that. You could go before a medical committee and say, 'Listen, that's as good as it was going to get,' and nobody could challenge you. But if you don't take the time, I'd say you have an ethical problem."

Some ethical problems go beyond specific cases and involve decisions that must be made by entire medical-bureaucratic systems.

Here are a few nonhypothetical problems:

Suppose a patient is suffering from hepatitis B, a wildly infectious blood-borne disease, or from AIDS. He also desperately needs abdominal surgery. In this kind of surgery, the surgeon often is working blindly, deep inside the body. In such circumstances, he may stick himself with hypodermic needles or nick himself with a scalpel. If he does this with a hepatitis-B or AIDS patient, he, the surgeon, could be infected. He could lose his life or his career. Is he ethically obligated to operate? The question is critical right now, with the appearance of AIDS and its growing impact on the medical-care system.

What are the ethical options for a rural hospital, perhaps the only one for dozens of miles around, when it finds that it doesn't attract quite enough cases to support itself? Should borderline cases involving elderly Medicare patients be "stretched" a bit, since most of the costs are borne by the government? Should doctors in small hospitals take a run at all cases that are not clearly beyond their means, rather than routinely transferring complicated problems to urban medical centers? Suppose the difference in money collections would mean the survival of the hospital, and that, in turn, might mean that dozens of other people over the years would survive heart attacks, automobile accidents, and other traumas. Would that make a difference?

What about that old favorite, the question of when to pull the plug? Should doctors take extreme measures to save someone who will certainly die later? Should an experimental heart technique be attempted with a baby who can't say no and who will almost certainly die anyway, after more days and days of intense pain? And would you say yes rather than no if you thought those painful, death-delaying techniques might someday lead to operations that would save the lives of other babies?

Just thirty years ago, heart bypasses were radical. Now they are routine. Five years ago, heart-lung transplants were thought to be an almost unimaginable goal. Now they can be done, but the goal wasn't reached without pain and death. Is the pain and death justified?

Ethical problems are pervasive. They're involved in everything doctors do. It has become something of a fashion for medical schools and hospitals to set up ethics committees to discuss the problems.

"The best thing you can hope for is awareness and honesty. But you can get crooks, guys who just don't worry about it, and then you've got trouble," Cunningham said.

Bad Results

IN EVERY surgeon's life there are cases with unsatisfactory results.

"Everybody has them," said Cunningham. "There's a whole two-volume study of unfavorable results, just in plastic surgery. You're not going to have them every day, but they're going to be there, and you have to deal with them."

Unsatisfactory outcomes are particularly devastating for plastic surgeons: they are, after all, doctors who specialize in *improvements*. Any unsatisfactory outcome is a serious defeat.

"If you take out a gallbladder and the wound gets infected and you have a healing problem, well, you manage it. At the end of the road, the patient's gallbladder is out and that's what you started to do. If you take a woman who wants a facelift, and she gets an infection, has problems with healing and winds up with scars, you've done exactly the opposite of what you started to do. You made things worse, not better," he said.

Legal considerations make it impossible for Cunningham to discuss specific cases in which he has had bad results. Given the aggressive presence of malpractice attorneys, physicians are wary of discussing individual problems without the closest legal advice. But the general situation—that all physicians have poor outcomes in some cases—is well known. Cunningham thinks public discussion is not only proper, but desirable.

"I don't think we should be embarrassed about talking about bad results. We should be honest about it, so the public gets it in mind that we're not all Marcus Welbys. This is a human profession and sometimes things go wrong," he said.

Unsatisfactory outcomes can be generally classified under four headings:

- The surgeon makes a judgmental or technical error before or during the operation, or while managing the recovery.
- The patient makes an error in managing the recovery.
- There is an "act of God."
- The patient is unhappy with the outcome, although the surgeon believes it is satisfactory and sees no error.

The most common medical complications of plastic surgery are hematomas (bruising) and infection. In most cases, they are easily managed—but either can get out of hand.

In serious hematomas, substantial amounts of blood may collect beneath the skin. That can place undue stress on suture lines, creating undesirable levels of scarring. With skin grafts and other operations, a spreading hematoma can destroy the tiny new blood vessels that are trying to establish themselves between the new skin and underlying tissue. As a result, the skin may die.

Infections can cause some of the same problems as hematomas—the swelling places stress on suture lines, or the infection may interfere with blood flow and cause tissue death. The treatments for both hematomas and infections are well known and of wide variety. The critical point is that the treatments be applied quickly.

Other problems are less common.

Prosthetic devices, such as breast-enhancement pads or chin

implants, can "migrate." That doesn't mean that they wander aimlessly around the body, but simply that they move a bit. Even a small motion in a prosthesis like a chin implant, however, can cause appearance problems—asymmetry, improper shaping, or an extended chin called "witches chin."

In very rare instances, implants can be extruded, which means that they force their way out through the skin.

Some operations can cause numbness of the skin. It happens frequently in forehead lifts and breast-reduction and shaping (mastopexy) operations. Facelifts can result in hair loss, scarring, or damage to facial nerves. An eyelid lift (blepharoplasty) can result in dry-eye syndrome, in which the tear glands do not produce sufficient lubrication for the eyes. And there have been cases of blindness as a result of uncontrolled infection. Rhinoplasties may produce unexpected bleeding, sometimes as much as two weeks after the operation. Breast enhancements can result in "capsules" of scar tissue around the implant, resulting in a "tennis ball" look. The anesthesia in an operation can cause a variety of problems, some extremely serious.

Surgeons make out-and-out errors: facial motor nerves have been cut in facelifts, resulting in paralysis of some facial muscles. Skin grafts have been placed upside down, in which position they inevitably die. Surgeons have been so intent in placing skin grafts that they neglect the graft donor site, which becomes infected, and which may later need a graft itself to close the now-serious wound. Poor selection of graft donor sites can lead to such undesirable effects as a growth of pubic hair on the hand. . . .

There are, in fact, hundreds of possible unfavorable outcomes for the dozens of different plastic surgeries, though none are common as a percentage of operations.

"There can be mistakes leading to unfavorable results from the time the patient walks in the door until you wave good-bye. There are critical points all the way through the relationship," Cunningham said.

Cunningham has begun doing increasing numbers of "revisions," which means he tries to fix unsatisfactory plastic surgeries done by other surgeons.

In that experience, he said, the classic surgical "oops"—a gross surgical mistake—is fairly uncommon. Usually the problems are ones of judgment, and even good surgeons make them.

"It's not usually the situation where the surgeon says, 'Gee, I wish I hadn't accidentally cut through the facial nerve' [while separating the skin from underlying tissue in a facelift]. Usually it's a situation where a guy is in a complicated rhinoplasty and he says to himself, 'You know, I think I can get another millimeter or two off that cartilage,' and it turns out that he couldn't. He puts the thing back together and it's lopsided, asymmetrical, or too small, and the patient becomes very unhappy."

Conceptual difficulties also occur. The surgeon thinks he knows what he's doing but does not. Cunningham said that plastic surgeons who work in overwhelmingly Caucasian areas, for example, often don't understand nose characteristics of other racial groups.

"You don't just take a quick look and understand the geography of a nose. A lot of people don't understand that the difference between a typical black nose and a typical Caucasian nose is that the black nose is smaller. You need to add onto it. You don't need to trim away at the cartilages at the tip to make the tip look smaller. So we see people coming in who have had those cartilages trimmed down and they're unhappy, and they should be. The surgeon didn't understand what was going on. Technically, he was okay. The knife didn't slip, he did what he wanted to do, but what he wanted to do wasn't the right thing."

Surgeons are not the only ones who can make errors that affect the outcome of a surgery. Patients make them, too.

"When I'm doing a facelift on a patient who smokes, I tell them they've got to quit for three weeks. Three weeks, or I won't do the operation. They'll have to go somewhere else."

He explained that there are areas behind the ear and on the neck that are a relatively long way from any powerful blood supply. The skin in those areas is supplied by small, delicate blood vessels. Nicotine acts as a vascular constrictor, narrowing their size.

"If you smoke, it could have the effect of choking off the blood supply—not so you'd notice normally, but so that it could cause trouble after the bruising and distress of an operation. If those blood vessels break down, you could wind up with ulcers in there, scabs, the whole thickness of the skin could die. You can tell that to people, and they'll swear with the best intentions that they'll quit. Then they don't. They can't stand it. That can get you into trouble."

The same thing can happen with breast-reduction operations, with the nicotine closing down the small blood vessels that lead to the nipple. If that happens, the nipple may die, leaving the patient with an open wound and a disfigurement.

Patients can also get into trouble by failing to follow preoperative or postoperative routines. If a patient is scheduled for a morning rhinoplasty, wakes up with a tension headache, and pops a couple of quick aspirins to control it, that simple act can have serious consequences. Aspirins thin the blood and make bleeding harder to control. That's not usually disastrous, but could force a surgeon into extra procedures, or to hurry the routine. If it's bad enough, he may have to order special blood studies and treatments to counteract the aspirin. At that point, he's doing damage control that should not be part of a routine rhinoplasty.

Other patients, told not to eat, become very hungry in the morning before their operation and decide to sneak "just a cookie." If the anesthetic nauseates them (a common complication) and they begin vomiting while only partially conscious, there is a danger that they might breathe in some of the vomit and choke.

Postoperatively, some patients insist on resuming strenuous exercise regimes too quickly, or, in the case of breast enhancements, fail to do scheduled massages. The self-massages reduce the possibility that scar tissue will encapsulate the silicone pads.

Weight gain can be a problem, especially for women who have

undergone procedures like mastopexies that reshaped their breasts. Too much new weight can result in the same gravity-generated slump that they suffered before the operation.

Too much sun can be a problem, further damaging skin that is already in shaky condition after an operation. And for some kinds of surgery, the patient has to be careful not to make motions that will cause blood pressure to surge, such as bending over too quickly.

Cunningham believes one of the biggest mistakes a surgeon can make is to allow the patient to believe that the surgery is not serious.

"You don't want to scare them to death. You don't want to lean forward and say, 'My God, you know you could get a shot of anesthetic and develop a heart arrhythmia and die right there on the operating table.' That's stupid. But they have to be aware that it's a serious business. For any given operation, you want to be very clear ahead of time about what can go wrong. You want to make it very clear that we both have responsibilities, and I'll take mine seriously but they've got to take theirs seriously, too."

The acts of God are another kind of problem.

A patient can be prepared for some of them. For others, there is no real preparation.

"Maybe ten to fifteen percent of the women who have breast enhancements are going to develop overly firm breasts—the scar tissue will form capsules around the pads—and in some cases we'll have to go back [and release the capsules with another round of surgery]. That just happens," Cunningham said. "You have to prepare the patient for the possibility. You don't want them coming in saying, 'Yeah, I understood that it happens to some people, but I didn't think you meant me.' That's bad news."

The other kind of act of God is more dangerous—it's the unforeseen, uncalculable situation. The tissue structures are not normal. Healing does not proceed normally. Bleeding can't be controlled. The patient has an unpredictable reaction to anesthesia or to drugs.

"Almost anything you can think of, we have procedures to deal with," Cunningham said. "It's very important, though, that the surgeon recognize that he's in trouble, that there's a problem, and that he can admit it. That takes time. I think it probably takes three or four years of working on your own, every day, before you can say, 'Okay, here's a problem, what are we going to do with it?' and really be confident that you can deal with it, whatever it is.

"I had a patient who had some work by another doctor, and she just wasn't healing right. She had an open wound, and they couldn't get it closed. After I got to know her a little bit she told me that she hated to go to this guy's office because his attitude was, 'How can you do this to me? How can you just not heal like this and cause me all this trouble?' Finally, after about a month— she was a timid sort—she finally got up the nerve to say, 'Listen, this is not my fault. I don't want this to happen to me.' And she left and she didn't go back."

Perhaps the most common of the undesirable outcomes are those in which the patient is dissatisifed, but the doctor can defend the work as aesthetically and technically acceptable. That tends to happen when the doctor did not fully understand what the patient wanted.

"That's poor communication and there are ways to deal with that. You just have to be very meticulous about learning what the patient wants. If you do that, you don't run into the situation where you think it's great, and she thinks it's terrible, unless there's a psychological problem of some kind."

When both the patient and the physician agree on what is needed but the patient is dissatisfied after the operation, the doctor usually knows what she's talking about. "What usually happens is that the patient comes in and is very straight about it. She says, 'Yeah, it's okay, but it's not quite the nose I wanted. Should I have this little bump here?' And the doctor, if he's honest and has a good relationship with the patient, will admit that it's not quite the nose he had in mind, either. Not that it's bad, but it's not quite what he wanted and he recognizes that it's not quite what the patient wanted. Then the question is, what are you going to do about it, and who is going to pay for it," Cunningham said.

Most plastic surgeons do touch-up operations for minimal fees, although the patient is expected to pay hospital bills. "Sometimes, you just wind up saying, 'That's the best I can do. It's not exactly what I wanted to do, but that's the best there is.' In that case, everybody winds up with a sour taste in their mouths. You don't like to see those."

Whatever the complication and its cause, it's essential that the surgeon have the right relationship with the patient. He must be scrupulous in the preliminary interviews in telling them what can go wrong and impressing them with the reality of these potential problems. At the same time, he must avoid unnecessarily frightening the patient.

When the complication does occur, he should have earned enough trust that the patient will help him deal with it.

"The worst thing you can do is get in some kind of high-volume deal, a patient comes in, you say, oh, you wanna look younger, get a facelift, here's my secretary, she'll tell you all about it. The secretary gives them the rap, tells them you're a great doctor. But then if something goes wrong, the patient has no relationship with you. And they won't be looking to the secretary to tell them what went wrong. You've got to have the kind of relationship where you can talk about the complication and the options that are open to you," Cunningham said.

In at least one state, the doctor-patient relationship and medical ethical standards are not considered sufficient to deal with the risks of poor outcomes.

Maryland has passed a law that requires plastic surgeons to provide a state-written pamphlet to prospective breast-reconstruction and breast-enhancement patients. The booklet outlines possible dangers in the procedures, including encapsulation, blood clots, infection, rupture of the implant, the possibility that silicone gel will bleed through the implant wall into surrounding tissue, changes in sensation in the breast, loss of sensitivity in the breasts, and possible difficulties with future breast X rays and breast self-examinations.

A number of Maryland doctors have argued that while the booklet's warnings may be generally accurate, they do not realistically portray the degree of risk involved. Some of the warnings relate to problems so rare that they are statistically insignificant (rupture of a transplant pad, for example) or unproven and unlikely (that the pads would interfere with mammography, or that dangerous silicone bleed takes place).

The booklet, which is required only for the breast operations, was mandated by the legislature after several years of lobbying by a consumer who had experienced a bad result with a breast operation.

Burns

PEOPLE FIND all kinds of ways to hurt themselves. A nurse at any metropolitan emergency room can recite a catalogue that sounds like a macabre advertisement for kitchen appliances: human beings are ground, chopped, puréed, sliced, diced, and mashed. People are shot, stabbed, speared, beaten, and slashed. They fall on ice and out of trees and barn lofts. And they are burned.

Of all the injuries inflicted on human beings, burning may be the worst. Burns are the most painful injuries and among the most disfiguring. They are common. Roughly twelve thousand Americans die each year from burns. Several times that number suffer serious burn injuries. Burns are sustained in gas explosions, house and office fires, automobile, industrial, and recreational accidents, and in electrical mishaps. Children are often hurt by scalding.

In the burn ward in a hospital, you can hear patients screaming in anguish. Talk to a person who has suffered a serious burn, and the talk will always come around to "the bath" where burned tissue is cleansed from the body. They universally describe it as the most painful experience of their lives.

A surgeon specializing in burns once said that patients are frequently bothered by the painkilling drugs they are given. The drugs slow the mind. The patients feel stupid, unable to track normal conversations.

"Quite a few of them ask that we lower the level of the drugs—they say they'll take a little more pain in exchange for a little less drugs. But then in a day or two, they ask to have the drugs back. The pain is too much. They'd rather have the foggy mind," the surgeon said.

Burns come in three, or sometimes four, degrees. First-degree burns involve only the outer layers of the skin—a common sunburn is a first-degree burn. Second-degree burns damage deeper layers of the skin, but not so seriously that the skin cannot regenerate itself. Second-degree burns are intensely painful, but usually heal in two or three weeks. Sometimes second-degree burns are so bad, however, that skin grafts provide better texture and better skin quality than grown-in-place skin.

Third-degree burns are extremely serious. The classic indication of a third-degree burn, often cited in first-aid books, is charring—the skin is burned black. Technically, third-degree burns are those that destroy the skin and its appendages, so that the burned skin cannot regenerate itself. Those burns must be covered with skin grafts or with skin moved over the burn from an adjoining area.

Some doctors classify extreme burns as fourth degree. These burns go beyond skin damage and involve extensive loss of other tissue—muscle, bone, or tendons.

Severe burns are essentially open wounds. They don't bleed because the blood vessels have been too badly damaged. As open wounds, burns are susceptible to massive infection. The only way permanently to prevent infection is to cover the burn site with new skin.

Not just any skin will do. The human immune system is designed to fight foreign elements in the body—bacteria and viruses, for example. It will also fight foreign tissue, including foreign skin, so skin grafts must be taken from the burn victim's own body. The wound may temporarily be covered with pig skin or skin from a cadaver, but eventually it is always rejected. The patient is left with the open burn wound.

Because of these problems, a person with a 100 percent third-degree burn will die, either immediately from shock or within several days from overwhelming infection. Persons with lesser burn coverage, in the range of 75 or 80 percent, may or may not survive, depending on age, physical condition, and other individual characteristics.

When a burn victim arrives at a hospital with an extensive but survivable burn, the doctors first try to stabilize his body functions. Then, almost immediately, they start a series of sophisticated antiseptic techniques to reduce the chance of infection. As soon as the patient can tolerate it, the skin grafts begin.

Good skin is harvested from unburned areas with a noisy device called a dermatome. It looks something like an electric sander but works like a sod cutter, lifting strips of skin from the body. It doesn't lift full thicknesses of skin, as that would be pointless— it would amount to covering a wound in one place by creating an equally severe wound somewhere else. The dermatome takes only the top layers of the skin, leaving behind enough of a base that the donor area can heal itself. Indeed, when burns are extensive, the same donor site may be used over and over again, healing between each new skin harvest.

When the burn is extensive, and the good skin limited, the skin is meshed. The meshing turns the thin strips of skin into a net that can be stretched over a larger area than can unmeshed skin. The holes in the mesh then fill in from the sides.

Skin grafts are not pretty, particularly when done on the face. Skin lifted from other parts of the body is coarser than facial skin, and there are pigmentation differences. Scars form along the seams of the grafts, and the graft area takes on a patchwork effect. When meshed grafts are used, the healed skin has a pebbly surface, like that of a football.

Bad as the aesthetic results may be, grafts are the only method currently available to cover a burned area with living, infection-resistant skin.

Because burns are so painful and so disfiguring, the most heart-breaking of burn patients are children. Children do not under-stand why there is so much pain and why the people in the hospital seem to make it worse with their interminable treatment and repeated operations.

Jill was seven years old, a first grader. Her dark eyes peer at the world from a cave where she tries to hide from the pain. They are the same eyes that peer from photographs of young victims of the Holocaust.

Jill was a victim of a private holocaust when she was six months old. An accidental explosion left both her and her mother badly burned. Jill suffered burns on her head, which destroyed most of her hair-bearing scalp, on one side of her face, on her back, and on her right side and right chest. She lost one ear, which was burned to a small nubbin, and one forearm, which was am-putated halfway between the elbow and the hand.

On the morning of this particular operation, the fear began tearing at her composure in the prep room. She had undergone multiple operations every year of her life and knew what was coming: she sat nervously in a chrome and plastic institutional chair (the kind made not to relax in, but to be easily cleaned), her lips turned down in a ferocious grimace. Her eyes darted around frantically as she looked for the surgeon.

A half-dozen nurses were in the prep room, and they all kept telling her what a big girl she was. She knew what that meant, too: somebody was about to hurt her. She was wrapped in a children's hospital gown, an incongruously cheerful affair with a picture of a happy bear with a red cross on his hat. She clutched at a big pink-and-green bunny rabbit with floppy ears as she waited.

The stump on her right arm protruded from the sleeve of the happy gown. Her scarred head was covered with a blue gingham bonnet, straight out of the nineteenth century, complete with a lace frill around the edge. Her father sat beside her, trying to comfort her.

In an earlier operation, Cunningham had placed an empty balloonlike plastic expander under the portion of scalp with the biggest clump of hair. Every week or so after the first operation, he would use a syringe to pump sterile saline solution into the expander. As the expander got bigger, the scalp stretched to accommodate it (just as stomach or thigh skin on obese people stretches to accommodate growing accumulations of fat). Eventually, the area of good, hair-bearing scalp got bigger.

This morning's operation would remove the expander and spread the expanded skin over scarred scalp. If all went well, Cunningham intended to reinsert the expander for another round of stretching.

When Jill saw Cunningham coming, she began to cry. He dropped down to his knees in front of her and said, "Aw, come on, Jill, you always do so well, huh?" She continued crying, old enough now to know that Cunningham was trying to jolly her along. A nurse got down beside Cunningham and said, "You're such a big girl to be having this," and she began to look at Jill's arm to find a good spot for the intravenous needle.

"Are you going to put in the IV?" she squeaked.

Jill knows all the medical terms, and through spasms of tears told Cunningham that she didn't like the anesthetic gas she had last time. "It makes my nose feel funny."

"Did it make you sick?" Cunningham asked.

She nodded through the tears.

Cunningham said, "Good, you help us when you tell us that," and stepped over to talk to the anesthesiologist.

As the anesthesiologist and nurses looked through Jill's chart—an inch-thick paper file full of forms from previous work—Cunningham left the room and a moment later came back with his briefcase. He popped it open and took out a Nikkormat camera with an electronic flash.

"Okay, Jill, I'm going to take some pictures," he said. "Could you go up and stand there against the wall?" Jill put down her bunny and walked to the wall, taking off the gingham bonnet. She had been through this before, too.

Jill's face and neck were covered with red, streaky scars. Her skin was rough, with a pebbly, washboard surface. The front of her head had two small islands of hair, the larger about half the size of a dollar bill. There was more hair on the back and sides of her head. It was worn long so it could be arranged to disguise as much of the baldness as possible.

The hair-covered area at the back of her head, just above the join with the neck, was grotesquely deformed by the expander. Stretched almost to twice its normal size, the hair-supporting scalp bulged into a large sausage-shaped clump, like a massive tumor.

With Jill against the wall, facing him, Cunningham said, "Okay, can we get a smile? C'mon, just a little teeny smile." She stopped sniffing for a moment, and a tiny smile crept onto her face. Cunningham teased her about it, and finally a real smile cracked through and he took the picture. He went on to take side shots and finally a back view.

"You have to document what you do so you can review progress," Cunningham said later. "If we can fix this, it might be a paper. God only knows how many people could use it."

When Cunningham finished with the photos, a nurse led Jill back to the chair and she clouded up again. The nurse moved in with the IV needle and she started sobbing, but the needle went in cleanly and with little apparent pain. It was quickly taped in place.

"I'm cold," Jill said between sobs.

"That's okay, we'll give you a blanket," a nurse said, and Jill said, "Daddy, Daddy . . . ," and then turned back to Cunningham and asked when she'd get the shots.

"No, you won't need any shots or anything. There won't be any shots this time," he said. He looked over at the anesthesiologist: "I've got to head back to the lounge for a minute, come and get me when she's ready, will you?"

As he walked out of the prep room, he looked back at the girl. "I couldn't do it if I had to do kids all the time," he said. "I don't think I could handle it."

Cunningham, like all surgeons, carefully guards his emotions as they relate to patients. Surgeons see too many people who are badly hurt to allow themselves to become depressed each time. That's why surgeons and other medical personnel can be found humming little tunes while they work over automobile accident victims, or laughing and chatting about social events a few feet from a person undergoing the most desperate kind of surgery. The same reactions can be seen in police officers, firemen, news reporters, social workers, and other people who see a lot of tragedy. Some identification with a patient is okay—too much is not. Too much identification may drive a worker from his profession.

The trouble with young patients is that they can be emotionally irresistible. Nurse burnout, for example, is endemic in wards that specialize in treating children with serious illnesses. Part of the problem, the nurses say, is the incomprehension on the child's face, and their own inability to explain to a young child what is happening, why he hurts so much.

A child can break down necessary walls.

As Cunningham sat in the lounge and reviewed the girl's charts, the nurses and anesthesiologist wheeled Jill into the operating room. They moved her from the hospital gurney to the narrow operating table and put a blood-pressure cuff on the stump of her right arm.

When they were ready, a nurse went to get Cunningham. He walked in, tying on a surgical mask. As soon as she saw him, Jill asked, "Are they going to give me a shot?"

"No shot, no shot," Cunningham said. A few seconds later the anesthesiologist produced a large syringe and Jill almost panicked, struggling to sit up. The circulating nurse held her down and Cunningham leaned over her and said, "We're not going to give you a shot, no shot. Watch this, watch this."

As Jill watched, the anesthesiologist stuck the big needle into a valve in the IV tube and pushed down the plunger. Jill looked at her in disbelief. No shot.

"See, isn't that nice, you don't get a shot. No shot," Cunningham said. "You're going to get sleepy now and take a nap, and your daddy will be there to see you. Your daddy will be there when you wake up. . . ." He continued on that theme until the anesthetic hit, and she folded back onto the table. Cunningham kept saying her name until she was gone: "That's okay, Jill, everything is okay. . . ."

As she went down, a monitor began to beep, showing a heart rate of 95.

There were at that moment four doctors in the room: Cunningham; the anesthesiologist, who was busy with her monitoring equipment; and two residents, who waited for instructions from Cunningham. A surgical tech and three nurses completed the crew.

The first problem was the configuration of the patient: she had to be lying face down on the table to fully expose the burned scalp. That position complicated the arrangement of her respiration tubing, which could not be allowed to kink or to put damaging pressure on the tissue of her throat. Cunningham described the exact position that he needed, and the anesthesiologist began working with the nurses to figure out what they would need to build a supporting structure of pillows and foam "donuts" beneath the girl.

"If you look here," Cunningham said, rolling Jill's head in his hands, "you can see that there's not much to work with up on the front of her head. Her previous doctor divided this one clump of hair into two clumps, hoping that we could spread it, but she's so badly burned that the hair is sitting almost on top of the [skull] bone. There just isn't any blood supply there. When we try to expand it, we get infection problems, and we had to give that up. So now we've just got these two little islands of hair out here, and they don't do much."

The anesthesiologist decided what would be needed to support the girl's body and asked the nurses to get it. One of the younger nurses said to Cunningham, "Gee, it's going to take longer to get her in position than to do the operation."

"Yeah, it could, really," Cunningham said seriously.

As the doctors stood around waiting for the necessary supplies, and a nurse taped the girl's eyes shut, one of the residents asked about Jill's breasts. Her breasts were as yet undeveloped, but when Cunningham gently pinched her left nipple, a bud of tissue showed behind it.

"The breasts develop out of this tissue behind the nipple here. It looks on this side like it should be normal, but on the other side . . ." He reached across her body and pinched the place where her right nipple would have been. Now there was nothing but grafts and scarring on the surface, but there was still a bud of tissue beneath it. "It feels like we might get normal development over here, but because of the scarring problems, [the breast] could be displaced upward. We'll have to do something with that later, most likely. One problem you get with this kind of scarring, these burns, is the tissue distortion."

The nurses accumulated sufficient donuts and pillows, and got ready to turn Jill on her stomach. Just before they did, the anesthesiologist attached an oxygen monitoring device to one finger of Jill's left hand.

Jill rolled easily. An adult can be difficult to roll because it's so hard to get a grip on unconscious patients without hurting them. And you can't just order up more movers, because there's not enough space for them to gather around the body. Jill, who was going into the skinned-elbow, skin-and-bones stage of childhood, went over as easily as a flapjack.

As they began to prop her with pillows and donuts, more burn damage was evident. There were extensive burned areas on her back, and her thighs were marked with pale rectangles where skin had been harvested for grafts.

When she was finally arranged on the table to Cunningham's satisfaction, the three surgeons went out to scrub. The anesthesiologist made final checks on all of her monitoring, IV, and respiratory connections, and the nurses began draping Jill's small body to keep it warm. When they finished, the girl was buried beneath a pile of blue drapes, with nothing protruding but the back of her skull. Because of the distortion caused by the expander, and the odd coloring of the grafts, her skull didn't look like what it was. It looked like a knee, perhaps, or a skinny hip.

The operation went quickly.

One resident, working under Cunningham's close direction, made an incision just above the buried expander, at the juncture between good, hair-covered scalp and bare, pebbly skin graft. The scalp bled profusely when cut, and Cunningham sealed each bleeder with an electric cautery.

Cunningham warned the resident not to approach the expander with the scalpel. He should finish the approach with the cautery, Cunningham said.

"If you finish the cut with the [cautery] it's easier to avoid damaging the expander," Cunningham explained. "You actually have to melt through it with the cautery; a knife will go through it before you know it."

At that moment, the resident cut through a minor branch artery at the back of Jill's head, and it squirted blood into the wound. "Let me get that," Cunningham said. "Where is it?"

One of the residents had pinched down the artery with a finger, and as Cunningham leaned forward with the cautery, he lifted his finger. The artery spurted again, and a strong, squirt-gun pulse of raw blood hit Cunningham squarely in an unprotected eye.

"Can you believe this?" he asked in exasperation. He went back to the girl and sealed the artery. That done, he turned to the surgical tech, asked for a gauze pad and a pan of saline solution, and washed his eye with a heavy flow of saline.

"Jeez, Jeff," he said to the resident as he returned to the table, "I thought I'd been relatively sympathetic about your residency, you know, and now you do this to me. . . . I mean, if I get AIDS, it's manslaughter. . . ."

"Yeah, I'm leaving for Fort Lauderdale anyway. I've got my Windsurfer," said the resident.

"I'll be in San Francisco General [known for its AIDS treatment programs] and you'll be out windsurfing," Cunningham complained.

They worked for another minute and Cunningham turned to the circulating nurse and said, "Could you go back through her records and see what her record of transfusions is—just look through the jacket there. I think you'll find it in the lab reports."

In the week before the operation, there had been front-page news reports of several medical personnel getting AIDS (Acquired Immune Deficiency Syndrome) through skin contact with contaminated blood. One nurse had been infected when blood squirted onto her face and hands, and into her mouth. A dentist had been infected when his bare hands apparently contacted contaminated blood in a patient's mouth.

"Everybody is a little paranoid," Cunningham had said the week before the operation on Jill. This was the first time he had come in unprotected contact with raw blood since the news reports, although contact was not uncommon. He was somewhat disturbed because there were numerous cases of persons contracting AIDS through blood transfusions in the early '80s, before AIDS screening began.

As the nurse began looking for transfusion records, Cunningham and the resident opened the incision and exposed the expander, a glass-clear plastic bag filled with saline solution. A short plastic tube sprouted from one end of the bag. At the end of the tube was a plastic disk about the size of a quarter. Altogether, it looked like a high-tech flower. The "flower" was a target valve through which the saline was injected. It was flower-shaped so that it could be easily felt through the skin.

Cunningham cut the valve free from its stem and used a vacuum to suck out the saline solution. With the pressure released, the expander collapsed like a leaking balloon and was easily slipped out through the scalp incision.

Setting the expander aside, Cunningham cut carefully around the newly stretched scalp, with its clump of good hair, until it could be flattened out. The expanded skin covered several square inches of previously bare scalp. The new patch of hair-bearing scalp was roughly triangular in shape.

"You know, I might chicken out here," Cunningham said after

a moment. "I was going to put that expander right back in, but I don't know. It might be a little tight. I might chicken out."

"Yeah, you could," said a resident. After a moment he added, "Chicken out, I meant."

"Cunningham, shaken by the contemplation of his fate as an AIDS victim, loses his nerve and chickens out of the operation," Cunningham said in a radio voice.

"Let's get this off here and see what happens," he said in his normal voice, touching the grafted area just above the good hair. The resident quickly cut around the indicated area, and then Cunningham took over, lifting the skin graft off her head as though he were peeling an orange.

"Could you save that for me?" he asked the surgical tech, handing her the triangular scrap of brown skin graft. "I might want to use it again. Pop it in some saline, will you?"

With the graft gone, Cunningham advanced the expanded hair-covered scalp over the open wound. It fit quite neatly.

"Shazam," said the resident.

"I don't know, maybe I won't chicken out," Cunningham said. "We've got a little more room here than I thought. . . ." After another moment of work, he decided to reinsert the expander. He fitted it under the loose scalp, cut a hole farther down her neck, and led the filling tube and target valve out through the hole. Then the scalp was sewn in place over the expander.

"The scarring on her face will soften up as she gets older," Cunningham commented after a few moments of silent sewing. He prodded at the scalp with a finger and turned to the resident.

"You see how this point [on the triangle of good scalp] is white? The blood supply is really crummy under there, but you can get away with it most of the time. That's something to note. It'll look crummy for a while, but then it'll start working. But right now, it looks really blanched."

They continued stitching. The nurse who had been going through Jill's records reported that the girl had apparently not had a transfusion in the past three years.

"Not all the records are here, she's got another file, but these go back three years. She's had other operations but she hasn't needed any blood. I can get those earlier records if you want."

Cunningham asked her if she would, and she made a note.

"The stats show that kids develop AIDS quicker if they're going to have it, if they're HIV-positive," the resident commented. HIV stands for Human Immunodeficiency Virus. "She'd show it before now, if it's been three years."

"Sounds right to me," Cunningham said.

When both he and the resident had finished sewing, Cunningham smeared the wound line with a Vaseline-like antibiotic and gave instructions to the resident to keep her overnight.

"If she has any problem with the scalp or expander hold her over the next night and I'll see her Friday," he said, peeling off his gloves.

As Cunningham bumped out of the operating room, he was asked how long he expected to work on the girl.

"Years," he said.

"Like how many?"

"Three, four, who knows? The technology may change, we may be working on her for the rest of her life."

Too many burn victims are hopeless cases from an aesthetic point of view. When he works on them, Cunningham knows going in that he is doing a salvage operation. There's no chance for an elegant save.

But not all cases are like that. One exception involved a teenager named Luke, who also suffered a scalp burn.

When he was rolled down the hallway to the operating room on the hospital gurney, he looked scared—most people do—but no burns were visible.

"It's on the back of his head," Cunningham said.

The nurses and anesthesiologist got him into the operating room, hooked to an IV, anesthetized, monitored, and onto his stomach.

The stomach roll was more complicated in Luke's case than in Jill's, because he was so much larger. The roll was done in two operations. First the nurses prepared the supports that would go under him and hold him in place. Then they gathered at the side of the gurney opposite the operating table and got their hands beneath him and heaved. The first heave went nowhere. The surgical tech, who was already garbed in a sterile gown and therefore could not help, asked if she should get more people. One of the nurses clambered onto the gurney where she could get a better angle on the kid's inert body and answered, in a Russian accent, "Nooo, ve are stronk vimmen like bools."

When they rolled him, there was a second of excitement when a resident's paging beeper went off, and everybody froze and looked at the monitoring equipment. It didn't sound exactly like a monitor—it was pitched differently and too loud—but it was something weird, and a nurse said tensely, "What the hell is that?" Then the resident spotted his beeper on a chair and turned it off.

Once Luke was arranged on the table, Cunningham used the surgical version of an ordinary safety razor to cut hair away from the back of his head. The defect disguised by the long hair was large and gross.

What had happened, the resident said, was that the boy had been hit by a car and pulled beneath it. He wasn't hurt seriously by the impact—he suffered a broken arm—but his head had been pressed beneath an exhaust pipe. The pipe was as hot as an iron, and the resulting burn was six inches long and two and a half inches wide. The burned area was actually divided in two by a small bridge of less-badly burned scalp, as if the boy had tried to turn his head away from the heat. One of the burned areas was oval, the other just off-round.

Luke had been burned a year before the operation. Initial care involved removing dead tissue, including the old skin, and covering the area with a skin graft taken from his thigh. When the graft healed, it left a large, hairless defect on the back of his head. Although Luke wore his hair long and tried to comb it over the defect, the burn was simply too big to be disguised. In addition, the grafted skin had assumed an undesirable quality. It might have looked fine on a leg, but as part of the scalp, it resembled the skin of a newly thawed roasting chicken.

At the urging of his aunt, Luke went to Cunningham to see if anything could be done. There was something, and it involved the same procedure Jill had undergone, the placing of an expander.

In the preliminary operation, Cunningham made two incisions, each about two inches long, on either side of the defect. Using a spatulalike tool, the scalp was freed from underlying tissue. Skin expanders were placed under the scalp on either side of the burn.

When the incision healed, Luke visited Cunningham once a week for two months. Cunningham would locate the daisylike target valve by feel, and inject 10 or 15 cc of sterile saline solution through the target into the expander. The target valve was self-sealing so the saline could not seep back out under the scalp.

"We'd inject enough saline that he would begin to feel some pain—we'd really get it tight," Cunningham said.

The operation began with Cunningham injecting into the scalp large amounts of a local anesthetic laced with the drug epinephrine.

That done, he and the resident took a few minutes to scrub, came back, and stood beside each other at the head of the table. The resident started by cutting around the edge of the skin graft. The chickenlike skin had adhered to the underlying tissue and had to be freed.

When the skin graft was off, and the bleeding stopped, the boy was left with a gaping hole in the back of his scalp. It was an ugly sight, even for a surgical wound, red with blood and subsurface tissue. The expanders had been buried under good hair-covered scalp, so Cunningham and the resident had to undermine the viable scalp to locate and remove them.

When they found them, Cunningham sucked saline out of the expanders with a syringe, and when they were sufficiently deflated, slid them from under the scalp.

"Is his mom out there?" the surgical tech asked casually.

"I don't know exactly what the situation is," Cunningham said. "I think he's living with his aunt."

"Aw, poor kid," the tech said, patting the sterile blanket that covered the boy's butt.

"Jeez, plastic surgeons have been reprimanded for less than that pat," Cunningham said, cocking his eyebrows at the tech.

"I'm allowed. I'm a mother," the tech said.

The remainder of the operation consisted of shaping the final wound, placing temporary drains, and closing it. When the last suture was in, the boy had complete coverage of the old defect with natural hair.

"His hair will be just a touch thinner [over the burned area], but he's got so much hair that I don't think that even a barber would notice. It'll be essentially invisible," Cunningham said.

Later, in the hallway, he remarked that Luke had been a particularly pleasant case because he was old enough to understand what was being done, because he was young and healthy enough to easily tolerate the operations, and because the final result was so good.

The operation did produce one unexpected event. The skull bone directly under the expanders felt slightly flattened to Cunningham's finger. "I haven't seen that before," he said at the time. Later, he said that the flattening wasn't dangerous, but it was good to be aware that it could happen.

"Expanders are pretty powerful little tools. They haven't been around too long, and we're just finding out what we can do with them," he said.

The operations on Jill and Luke are fairly typical of Cunningham's burn work. Though most of the burn work performed by plastic surgeons is done after burns have been stabilized, they are occasionally involved in surgery with fresh burns.

One of the immediate problems that occurs in the wake of a serious burn is the development of an eschar, a leathery patch that forms over the burn site. The eschars are inflexible. If the burns go all the way around an extremity like a finger, leg, or arm, the inflexible eschars will resist the natural swelling that takes place after a burn. As the soft tissue beneath the eschar continues to swell, and the eschar continues to resist, pressure begins to grow beneath the burn. Sometimes the pressure can shut down underlying blood vessels, leading to gangrene and the loss of the extremity. If a large eschar is on the throat, doctors must carefully watch for signs that the windpipe is being compressed.

Plastic surgeons are often asked to cut through the eschars to release them and allow the burn site to expand along the incisions. (In the third-degree burns that produce eschars, the nerves are usually destroyed and no anesthetic is necessary to do the operation.)

Burns are intensely painful. Most big-hospital burn units provide psychological counseling to help patients deal with the stress of the pain and with flashbacks. The flashbacks, which can be triggered by the most mundane of events—television commercials, staring strangers, offhand comments from a spouse—carry the victim back to relive the agony and fear of the accident. The flashbacks can be psychologically devastating, making it impossible for a patient to work, play, or even sleep.

Counseling is also needed to help people deal with aesthetic problems. But that, say the patients, takes time and doesn't always work.

One young man in a St. Paul counseling group had his upper arms severely burned in an industrial accident, and lost much of his biceps muscles. Although he was notably good-looking in a cowboy style—broad shoulders, square chin, pale eyes—the scarring of his arms made it difficult for him to deal with women.

"I go out and things get going, and I get the feeling we're going to be going home together, and I say, 'You know, what you see is not exactly what you get,' and then I tell them about my arms. . . . Yeah, it really does turn some of them off. There's this one girl from the college, a really good-looking lady, she called me up for my birthday and said, 'Hey, let's do something,' and she doesn't seem to mind. But you know, who knows what people are thinking? It can really get on top of you, thinking

157

about it—and with me, it's my arms, and I can cover it with a shirt. What if it was like some people, and it was my face? I don't know if I could deal with that. That would really freak me out. As bad as I got it, I can stand here and say that I really couldn't tell you what must be going through their heads."

Cunningham offers no answers for that particular agony.

"All we can do is try to get better techniques. Maybe if we develop transplant therapy, we could do something. But I don't know. Sometimes, what you see is what you're going to have to live with, and there's not much more you can say. You give them the counseling and hope for the best," he said.

Snapshot: AIDS

The most controversial topic in the operating room in this decade is AIDS—Acquired Immune Deficiency Syndrome. At first seen primarily as a threat to homosexuals and drug addicts, by mid-1987 the disease was regarded as a major problem for the American health-care and medical-insurance systems.

Leaving aside the problems of the insurance system, some AIDS experts had begun to wonder whether the medical complex, which is highly labor-intensive, could stand up to the publicity given the deadly blood-borne affliction.

"It's not AIDS that's going to kill us, it's the fear of AIDS," said one authority on the disease. There are thousands of contacts every day between medical personnel and AIDS carriers. So far, less than fifty medical people have contracted the disease through their jobs after several million contacts. Even so, fear of the disease and uncertainty about the rate of infection are causing some critical but lower-level (and lower-paid) medical people to leave the field—nurses, laboratory technicians, paramedics.

The danger of the disease is most strongly felt in large metropolitan areas with significant populations of homosexuals and drug users, and in hospitals with large numbers of charity and emergency cases.

Those hospitals are particularly at risk because they routinely deal with drug users brought in by police, and because they are the first choice for delivery of serious trauma cases. In trauma cases, extensive surgical work often must be done without blood studies for the AIDS virus, or even the opportunity to ask the patient if he or she has tested positive for the AIDS virus. (AIDS bearers are termed "HIV-positive." HIV stands for Human Immunodeficiency Virus.)

One surgeon—not Cunningham—ticked off the problems on his fingers: "First, the population of HIV-positives may be one percent or more of the population. Second, there are studies that show the high-risk AIDS groups are also high-risk groups for other trauma care, so HIV-positives are probably overrepresented among the people brought into an emergency room. Third, the high-risk groups are overrepresented in big metropolitan areas as a percentage of the population. So what does that mean? That three or four or five percent of the people coming in covered with blood are HIV-positive? I don't know. I don't know what the risks are." He added that other studies, not directly related to the AIDS work, suggest that as many as 25 percent of sterile operating gloves come out of the OR with holes or leaks of some kind. "That's a little scary," he said.

Yet another surgeon said he was more worried about the other health professions than he was about surgeons themselves.

"I don't think the risk is that big, and I don't think doctors are going to stop operating on people. There's too much in the profession that says we keep working. But I'm worried about all the support people, the nurses and the orderlies and the lab technicians. We [surgeons] get paid the big bucks, but how many people are going to work in an emergency room for five or six bucks an hour? Or ten or fifteen bucks an hour, and not many nurses make that. . . . If these people get scared and start bailing out, the system is in trouble."

During the eighteen months of reporting for this book, table talk in Twin Cities operating and emergency rooms evolved from occasional theoretical discussions to deadly serious ethical arguments. Nervous jokes became the order:

. . . So the doc comes back in and tells the guy he's got AIDS. And the guy says, "Oh, no, doc. What can you do for me?" And the doc says, "Well, the first thing I can do is change your diet. We're going to put you on pizza, flounder, and pancakes." And the guy says, "Pizza, flounder, and pancakes? Is that really going to help?" And the doc says, "No, but those are the only things we can slide under the door."

During the spring and early summer of 1987, there were several reports of health-care workers getting AIDS from accidental contact with AIDS-contaminated blood.

"A lot of plastic surgeons are speculating on what we would do if confronted with an AIDS case, but most of us haven't been confronted with it yet. I personally don't think there is a role for aesthetic surgery for somebody who has tested HIV-positive," Cunningham said one day. "I don't think you can justify purely elective surgery, given the risks to the surgeon, the nurses, the techs, and the people on the ward."

Cunningham figured that he cuts himself or sticks himself with a needle once or twice a year, but said it happens more often to other surgeons, who are working in less ideal circumstances.

"I was talking to another surgeon here at the university, a guy who does a lot of work deep in the abdomen. You can't see in there as well as you can see with our plastic surgery, you get really cramped, and he said he gets stuck once a week or once every couple of weeks. I think that kind of thing is more common than we recognize," he said.

There are already some surgeons who would decline to work on an AIDS victim no matter what the circumstances, Cunningham believes.

"Most of us feel an obligation to work on people in health-saving or lifesaving situations—there aren't many people who would turn somebody down in a case like that, but I think there might be a few. It is absolutely necessary for us to know who does test HIV-positive, so we can take precautions, we can know what we're getting into. And there might be a few rural or community hospitals that simply wouldn't have the facilities or the training to deal surgically with somebody who had an infectious disease like AIDS. They might find it necessary to refer to other places where they do have the facilities."

Many surgeons have begun wearing special operating goggles to reduce the possibility of being squirted in the eye by blood from a severed artery, as happened to Cunningham while working on the young burn patient. And there is talk of specially armored operating gloves to protect against penetration by hypodermic needles or scalpels. Those, however, are not yet generally available.

Cunningham says that one of the biggest barriers to better protection of the health-care system is politics.

"Different social and medical groups are at different stages of discussion about this thing. A lot of medical people, especially in frontline cities like San Francisco and New York, are terribly paranoid about male patients, with some justification. We're pretty frontline here, and we're starting to get worried ourselves.

"But with some groups, the discussion still involves privacy and other legal issues. I went to a [plastic surgery] meeting and one of the people from a big urban center said that he was going to start requiring [AIDS blood studies] from all gay-appearing men before he'd work on them. But somebody said that would be illegal, that he'd have to make it all men, or maybe everybody, or it would be discrimination," he said. "We just really don't know what the legalities are right now."

Cunningham's wife, Marie, who is also a plastic surgeon, had a personal close encounter with the AIDS virus in a way that left her frightened and angered, Cunningham said.

"She was asked to see a patient in the emergency room, who'd cut his finger. She went to see him without even thinking about it—we're more aware of AIDS now, and a lot of people routinely pull on a glove before they'll even get close to a bleeding patient. Anyway, it was a bloody wound, and she took off the dressing and worked on it, then later she put on some gloves and [closed the wound].

"Later, the guy came back in for more surgery, and somebody asked him if he had any other illnesses. He said, 'Oh, yes, I'm HIV-positive.' Marie heard about it and she went berserk. She called the internist who asked her to work on the guy, and she said, 'You sonofabitch, what's going on here? Why didn't you tell me he was HIV-positive? I would have still worked on him, but I would have gone about it differently.'

"And this physician retorted that this was private and confidential information. Now I think that is a totally unacceptable, criminal viewpoint. If the individual had hepatitis, the medical staff would be routinely told so they could take logical precautions.

"There is no confidentiality issue here. There just isn't. If you've got it, you've got it, and the [hospital staff] should know about it so you don't destroy somebody else's life or the whole health-care system. Having other people know about it might have an unfortunate impact on the individual with AIDS, but for the other people, it's a survival issue, not just a privacy issue."

In the summer of 1987, the federal Centers for Disease Control in Atlanta recommended that hospitals augment a procedure called universal controls. All patients would be treated as if they have AIDS, when there is any possibility that medical personnel will come in contact with the patient's blood or other body fluids. Doctors, nurses, paramedics, and other technical people would wear gloves for all contact where body fluids may be present and may also go to increased use of gowns, masks, and goggles.

A doctor involved in hospital disease control said that the universal controls were overdue: "Some hospitals were already moving in this direction before AIDS ever showed up. Hepatitis-B kills more medical people than AIDS ever will, it's much more infectious, and the universal controls were needed to cover that problem.

"It will, however, take extensive training, and may still meet resistance," he said.

"There'll be two kinds of resistance. The first kind will be the people who think it's ridiculous to take these precautions with everybody. You get a bleeding kid, why put on a glove? But we know there are kids with AIDS. Still, some people will be philosophically opposed on the grounds that the universal protections put another barrier between the doctor and the patient, and that most of the time it's unnecessary.

163

"The second kind of resistance will come from people who will think this is a dodge to keep the identities of AIDS patients a secret. That's one of the big controversies—if a guy's got AIDS, should everybody know? Should he be labeled in some way? If we use and enforce universal protections, it might not be necessary to tell everyone in the hospital, as long as the people involved in the treatment know about it. But some people would say that AIDS should be a public matter, at least within the medical community. That everybody should know.

"Even if you take that view, though, you still need the universal controls. At least, I think so. If a guy comes in from a car accident and he's bleeding all over the place and you've got to get into him quickly, you're not going to have time to do the blood studies. That's when you've got to have universal protection techniques in place."

Asked about the doctor to whom Cunningham referred—the surgeon who frequently works blind, guiding instruments with his fingers, and therefore often sticks himself with needles or nicks himself with scalpels—the disease-control specialist shook his head.

"I don't know. I don't know what you do in those cases. You could suggest that they double-glove, but there have been studies that show that double-gloving doesn't really offer much protection. Some of the surgeons would have trouble with that anyway, because they need the sensitivity you get with thin gloves. . . . I don't know what we do."

He added, however, that the actual concentration of AIDS viruses within the blood is very low, and that in most instances of minor sticks or nicks, not enough blood would be transferred to give the surgeon the disease. But there are no guarantees, either.

As the hospitals began to stir with the debate over AIDS controls, national attention focused on a Minneapolis trial in which a jail inmate, an AIDS carrier, was tried for assault with a deadly weapon because he bit jail guards.

He was convicted.

"I don't know if you can pass AIDS on in saliva, but that's the way the culture is going to start viewing these things. It's going to be very hard on the AIDS victims, but we have to provide some protection to people who work with them. That's for everybody's good, including the people with AIDS," Cunningham said.

Breast Reconstruction

AESTHETIC SURGERY has long been controversial, even in medical circles. The controversy is inevitable. Plastic surgeons deal in matters as nebulous as beauty and perform costly, sometimes painful operations not demonstrably needed to improve the physical health of the patient.

In recent years, the controversy abated as the broader effects of plastic surgery became more apparent. There has even been a growing consensus that some operations, labeled "aesthetic" in the past, may be more accurately designated as functional repair. The distinction is not academic: group medical insurance policies pay for functional repairs. They do not pay for purely aesthetic surgery.

The revision of opinion has been sharpest in regard to breast operations. Consider the example of the woman who cannot jog or take part in other normal, relatively mild sports because of excessively large breasts. More and more surgeons will argue that she's as effectively handicapped as a person who has lost a foot. The psychological abuse visited upon a woman with extraordinarily large breasts might well be considered an additional handicap.

Breast reconstructions, in which a surgeon creates a new breast to replace a breast lost to cancer surgery, also were considered aesthetic surgery at one time. Mastectomy patients do not need breast reconstructions for physical health reasons. And the loss of a breast can be disguised with clothing: the mastectomy patient will not be shunned on the streets. Still, the motives for undergoing a breast reconstruction are anything but trivial. Breast operations of all kinds deeply engage the feminine psyche. That is particularly true in the case of a breast lost to cancer, where the scarred chest is a constant reminder of a brush with death.

An astonishing number of women undergo mastectomies each year. Each must decide whether or not to undergo reconstruction.

"I can't give you any typical reason that people have reconstructions," Cunningham said. "You can get a hundred different answers. But if I were going to boil it down, I think these women want to feel whole again. They want to feel healed. They want to get the cancer behind them. People who don't have reconstructions—I don't know why they don't. Fear, maybe. They've had enough of hospitals and doctors and surgery, and they want to get away from it. You could get about as many reasons as you have people."

Results of reconstruction operations are generally good. The new breasts (and new nipples, if the patient chooses to have them) are reasonably natural. Like rhinoplasties, breast operations come in different degrees of complication. Some are not much harder than breast enhancements. Some involve the most delicate of microsurgical techniques.

At the simplest level are reconstructions after subcutaneous mastectomies, which are performed on women who show precancerous changes in breast tissue, but no actual cancer. In these cases, the breast tissue—fat and gland—is removed, but the underlying muscles, the skin, and the nipples are left intact. Reconstruction involves the placement of a silicone breast implant beneath the skin, much as is done in a breast enhancement.

Reconstructive procedures become dramatically more difficult as the mastectomies become more radical and more and more skin and muscle is removed.

In early 1986, Cunningham became seriously interested in an operation on a woman who had had a radical mastectomy two decades earlier. Although considered necessary at the time, the technique used is now considered somewhat excessive in most cases. The operation removed not only her right breast, but also the underlying chest muscle, the pectoralis major. There had been no attempt to build a new breast. The wound left by the mastectomy had been covered by a skin graft. The graft lay directly on top of the ribs, and had become attached to the rib bones.

Now the patient was asking for a reconstructed breast. To build a new breast, Cunningham would have to find new muscles to replace those the earlier surgery had removed, to serve as a support for the implant.

To get those muscles, Cunningham proposed to cut free most of a large back muscle, the latissimus dorsi. It starts near the back of the armpit and covers much of the midback below the shoulder blades. When the muscle was free, he would tunnel beneath the skin on the woman's side and chest, and insert the back muscle where the chest muscle had been.

The operation is called a "flap," which means that tissue is moved from one place to another but critical blood vessels are left intact. ("Free flaps" are operations in which tissue is cut completely free from the body and transplanted elsewhere. In those cases, new blood connections are made.) Flap operations involve some risk because of their complexity. The muscle is almost totally removed from its natural bed, and almost all blood connections are severed. If the remaining vessels are not big enough to supply sufficient blood (and the size of vessels may vary from patient to patient), then the muscle will die. Infection can be a problem, as can excessive bleeding—and either can result in the loss of the flap.

After several detailed examinations and a long discussion, the woman elected to go for the reconstruction and was scheduled for surgery.

The operation was at University Hospitals: green tile walls, speckled terrazzo floors, stainless-steel cabinets full of drugs with names like dexamethasone, Dobutamine, atropine sulfate. A jazz flute played in the background, breathy, arrhythmic, scratching through the speaker of a radio.

All of the hospitals where Cunningham works have distinct personalities. One, a small community hospital, is friendly and even chatty. The nurses and anesthesia people all know one another and have worked together for years. Every once in a while, Cunningham will be absentmindedly called "dear" or "honey" by the middle-aged nurses. At a big metropolitan medical center where he works, the atmosphere is much brisker and even cynical: the people there have seen everything and will not allow themselves to show surprise or shock. They are the pros. They do what needs to be done.

University Hospitals has more of a teaching atmosphere, even through many of its operations are purely routine, nonteaching matters, with neither students nor residents present. Still, the instructional background gives the place a more formal, much cooler attitude. Bureaucratic rules are more rigorously applied, procedures followed without exception, even when the exceptions would make sense.

This operation began with a lengthy conference on the placement of the patient. For the first part of the operation, she would be on one side, facing slightly down. For the latter part, she would be on her back. The process was carefully outlined for the anesthesia and nursing personnel until everyone understood.

After all the talk and mental rehearsal, the operation began like all of them, when Cunningham asked the surgical technician for a knife and she handed over a scalpel.

The woman was asleep, her eyes taped shut, her breathing steady and deep. She had been placed three-quarters facedown, with her right shoulder blade pointed up. Cunningham took the scalpel, placed it at a likely starting point below the shoulder blade, and drew it across her back. A red line followed behind it, as though he was drawing with a red ballpoint pen. The first incision arched up, the second arched down, meeting at the ends. The incisions isolated a football-shaped island of flesh. When Cunningham completed the second incision, the wound gaped open. Translucent amber fat cells winked from the cuts.

There were three people huddled over the woman on the table, united in the anonymity of surgical gowns, masks, and hats. Cunningham did the cutting as the assisting resident held the wound open with retractors. The surgical tech passed instruments to both of them.

As Cunningham moved deeper into the wound, he exposed first a layer of fat, three-quarters of an inch thick, and then the red-purple bundles of working muscle. Blood began to flow heavily into the incision.

"Let's get in there with the Bovie [cautery]," Cunningham said and suggested that the resident try it.

"Thank you," the resident said, pleased with the trust implicit in the decision.

Cunningham, wielding two small stainless-steel rakelike instruments, pulled the edges of the wound apart and the resident began cutting and cauterizing. As each blood vessel was severed, it spouted blood until hit by the cautery. With each hit, the cautery made a sharp *zzzt*, like an insect hitting an electric bug-killer. Each *zzzt* was accompanied by a puff of smoke, and the operating room was quickly suffused with the smell of burning blood.

"Ah, if you could just suck some smoke there," Cunningham said to the surgical tech. "It'd make us all feel a little better."

The tech turned on a small vacuum and held its suction tube over the wound.

"Better," Cunningham said.

Cunningham, when operating, works intently through the hard patches and tends to talk during the easier parts—his way of relaxing.

"You have to relax sometimes. I mean, when you just can't,

you walk out of the operating room with this devastated feeling. Most operations, you find spots to relax, even when you're in really deep."

The talk comes in spurts, and now he said, apropos of nothing in particular, "She'll look a little flatter in the back, and will lose some function in the sense that she won't be quite as strong in the motion you'd make for an overhead serve or a butterfly [swimming stroke]. With this particular patient, that motion is not of major consequence."

The muscle-replacement operation was not unique, but it was not common, either. It faced one critical moment.

A large muscle like the latissimus gets blood from several separate sources—mostly small arteries, but also a few large ones. The primary blood supply to the muscle comes through a narrow neck of the muscle that extends up into the armpit.

It was just possible that the original radical mastectomy damaged the arteries in the armpit area. If it had, the other, smaller arteries had picked up the slack, and the muscle continued to function. That's called compensation, and it's a reasonably common situation.

But in dissecting out the muscle, Cunningham would be cutting all those subsidiary arteries. If the primary arteries had been damaged by the earlier operation, the muscle would have no good blood supply at all.

There were indications that the primary blood supply was working, but there was no practical way to know for sure without removing the muscle.

"So you find out at the very end whether the whole thing is going to work," Cunningham said. He wiggled his eyebrows over the blue surgical mask and continued in a fake Transylvanian accent: "Zat, my friend, is what makes zees operation zo interesting."

The latissimus was quickly exposed, with Cunningham and the resident peering under the woman's skin like a couple of kids might look at their feet under a sheet.

Cunningham: "Boy, she's bleeding a lot."

Resident: "Yeah, there's a good blood supply back there somewhere."

Cunningham to nurse: "You have another unit [of blood] on order?"

Nurse: "Yeah, you want another?"

Cunningham: "I don't think we'll need it, but you better check."

The nurse checked a list on a clipboard and called the hospital's blood bank with an operating-room telephone. The nurse at the bank assured her that the blood could be ready in minutes.

As the work on the breast reconstruction continued, most of the actual cutting was done by the resident, with Cunningham giving inch-by-inch supervision.

Cunningham: "See, right there, the lat slides under the trapezius [the large muscle that covers the upper shoulder, runs up the neck and down the center of the back around the upper spine; the stiff-neck muscle]. You have to be really careful separating them so you don't damage the trapezius. So here's the posterior side of the muscle right there, and we have to get it up fairly close to the humerus, and we're getting there. What we want to do is define the plane I'm on right here, see where I've got my finger under here? Put your finger right here where mine is. Feel that?"

The resident felt around in the wound.

"Yeah, yeah, I feel it."

The two men were tugging on the layer of fat and skin with one hand each, while probing with the fingers of the other. Surgeons often handle flesh in ways that seem simply . . . rude. It's obvious even to a layman that they're not doing damage, but when they have to know something, they are not shy about stretching out a piece of tissue and really looking at it, squeezing, probing, rubbing, moving lights to get a better look at it. There is no such thing as squeamishness.

Cunningham and the resident, digging with their fingers, worked out the exact lay of the muscle so they could separate it from underlying tissue. Cunningham helped retract, and the resident started in again with the scalpel and the cautery. A moment later, a sudden freshet of blood spurted into the wound.

172

"Ooo, look at that one," said the resident. He zapped the bleeder with the cautery.

Resident: "Missed. Where is it?"

Cunningham: "Right there."

Resident: "Right there?" Zap.

Cunningham: "Nope—right here, see, there it is." Zap.

Resident: "Okay, I got it."

Eventually the muscle was free, except for the small neck that runs under the armpit. Cunningham took the muscle in his hands and turned it, looking for the blood supply.

"It looks good," Cunningham said. He pointed to two small white lines in the slender neck of muscle. "You see that? That's the blood supply coming in. It looks fine."

In the next few minutes, Cunningham and the resident tunneled under the skin of the woman's side and chest, working from back to front under the arm. When the excavation was large enough, the loose latissimus muscle with its football-shaped island of skin was literally stuffed under the skin of the chest, like a sock under a T-shirt. It made a fist-sized lump about where the new breast would eventually be.

That done, they began closing the back wound, their hands and fingers weaving arabesque figures over the wound as they stitched it shut. The first step in the closing was done with heavy thread, and a half-dozen ties were made down the length of the wound. With the wound roughly closed, finer thread was used in a long running stitch to pull the incision into a neat line.

"I've become more convinced over the years that some people just do some stuff better than others," Cunningham said much later. "Their sensory input is stronger. The control they have of their fingers is better. And their intellect is more adroitly applied in these situations. I'm pretty good at things like wound closure. If you come watch a couple of residents close a wound, with me helping, you'll see an acute difference between what I can do, having done it for ten years, and what they can do. But you'll also see an acute difference between two residents, both with about the same amount of experience. One can simply do it better. That tends to even out over the years, but still, years later, the guy who was more adroit to begin with will still do it better. It's not a disgrace if you're less adroit—you just don't have the same disposition. You're probably better at something else."

This particular resident was slower than Cunningham, but was clearly quicker and more skillful than others with whom Cunningham had worked. As it happened, this resident was something of a favorite. Cunningham had hinted broadly on a couple of occasions that he might make a good plastic surgeon.

Cunningham also went out of his way to explain small technical points. There was, for example, a minor complication in closing the ends of the wound. Since the wound was football-shaped, the skin, when pulled together, pursed at the ends.

"You take out those dog-ears like this," Cunningham told the resident. He made a deft cut with a small scalpel, removing a Pac-Man shaped piece of skin from each end of the wound. That done, the wound closed smoothly and cleanly.

"It's a big wound," Cunningham said as he sewed. "If there's too much pressure on it, if you have to pull it too tight, you can have a problem with the healing. So you can't take too much [skin] or you're in trouble."

Skin, he added, stretches easily and naturally, and removing a chunk as large as a woman's hand will not limit movement if it's given a short time to heal and stretch.

The woman would have a substantial scar where the skin and muscle were removed. Cunningham oriented the incisions to minimize the scarring, but any cut that goes through the full thickness of skin will leave a scar.

"You have to ask, is it more unsightly to have a scar on the back? Or not have a breast? The patient has to answer that question. If she decides she wants a breast, there are some things we can do to minimize the scar, but you can't avoid it altogether. It's going to be there."

Time will also obscure the scar, he said, eventually leaving a white line, like a piece of string, across the patient's back.

The woman had been lying three-quarters facedown, her right shoulder and side propped up while the muscle was being dissected out. When the back wound was fully closed, she was gently rolled onto her back.

She was a thin, middle-aged woman, with high cheekbones and graying hair. Her one remaining breast was small and firm, and the firmness seemed to emphasize the absence of the other breast. The missing breast had been replaced with a skin graft the diameter of a cue ball. The graft was the color of old parchment, and tight, resembling the skin on a tambourine. The graft was directly on top of the rib cage, since the underlying muscles had been removed. In places it had attached itself to the rib bone. It was brutally efficient, and totally ugly.

Cunningham made a quick circular incision just off the edge of the graft and carefully peeled it away from the underlying bone. The lat muscle and the island of skin from the woman's back had been stuffed under the good chest skin just to the side of the graft. With the graft gone, Cunningham fished under the chest skin with his fingers and pulled out the replacement skin and muscle.

He laid the muscle out in a fan shape, with the big edge of the fan toward the center of the chest. If the new muscle and skin were simply sewn in place, the patient would have a tight, flat chest, and not much that would resemble a breast. Fortunately, both skin and muscle stretch easily. Expanders, like those used to expand the burn patients' scalps, can be used to make room for breast implants.

In the breast reconstruction, Cunningham used an expander that looked like a plastic ice pack—a disk-shaped plastic bag with a circular "lid." The "lid" was the target for a hypodermic needle.

"We put this under the flap [the skin and muscle] and after it [the wound] is healed enough, we'll inject saline solution into the bag with a syringe. You can feel this top part [the lid] through the skin, and that's your target. When we do the flap, she loses the nerves in this area, so she won't feel anything at all from the syringe," Cunningham said.

By increasing the amounts of saline in the bag every few days, both the skin and the muscle are stretched. When they're stretched enough, a permanent implant is placed beneath it. The permanent implant, like those used in breast enhancements, is a disk-shaped plastic bag filled with clear liquid silicone. Once buried under the skin, it closely simulates the heft and fluid qualities of a natural breast.

With the expander in place, the closing of the chest wound was routine—the muscle was tacked into place and would eventually develop further connections to the underlying tissue. While at first it would depend on the blood supply coming through the armpit area, additional small blood vessels would also grow into the muscle.

After the muscle was placed, Cunningham reshaped the chest incision to conform more closely with the skin taken from the back. The wound was finally closed with fine surgical thread. The skin color-match, from back to front, was virtually perfect.

When the wound had healed, and the artificial breast implant was done, the woman would have a breast-sized "bump" on her chest. In a bathing suit or brassiere, it would resemble a natural breast. It would have no nipple or the pink-toned areola around the nipple.

Building a nipple and an areola complex is no particular problem. It can be done quickly and simply, using pieces of reddish skin from the groin area. That operation would wait until the implant operation was completed and the wounds healed.

"I don't know if this patient will want that. Some do, some don't," Cunningham said. As he put the final few stitches in the reconstruction, he explained that some women are satisfied with breasts that look natural in social situations—swimming, or in thin clothing like tube tops—but are not particularly interested in going through the additional trauma of a nipple and areola reconstruction.

When he finished suturing the flap of skin and tissue in place, Cunningham stepped back from the table and nodded to the resident.

"That looks pretty good," he said, stripping off his gloves. He gave instructions for the woman's postoperative care, left her in the resident's charge, and headed to the locker room.

As he changed into his street clothes he said he was about to do another breast reconstruction. The woman having it done was "very articulate. She did a lot of research on it when she found out she had cancer." He suggested she could provide a good patient-view of the operation.

The woman, as it happened, was a lawyer for the state of Minnesota. In 1983 she found a lump in one breast during a self-examination.

"I didn't do the self-exams every month like you're supposed to, but I did them regularly," the woman said. "When I found it, it was relatively large, marble-sized or a little bigger. It was real obvious—I knew immediately I was dealing with a lump in my breast."

She went to her HMO and had a needle biopsy, which is an attempt to draw fluid from the lump. If fluid is present, it may indicate a cyst, rather than a tumor. No fluid was found, and she went to a surgeon for a full biopsy.

"I waited there, I was in the room when the phone call came back from the lab. I'd done all this research on what a biopsy involved, and I had kind of reassured myself. The doctor said I didn't fall into the cancer risk groups and so on, and I really didn't think I had cancer. I was just worried about how scarred I would be from the biopsy. . . . Anyway, the phone call came in and I heard him say, 'Really,' kind of surprised, and I knew that was a bad sign.

"When he told me I had cancer, I cried. That was an immediate reaction, and then I pulled myself together and went home and thought about it, what I wanted to do."

What the doctor recommended, and what she eventually decided to do, was to have a modified radical mastectomy. She had follow-up chemotherapy when it was determined that the cancer had spread to the lymph nodes.

"I was one of the lucky ones with the chemotherapy," she said.

"It made me a little bit sick, but not too bad, and I didn't lose my hair."

The following year, just as she was finishing the chemotherapy, early signs of cancer were found in her other breast, and it, too, was removed.

By the summer of 1984, she was recovering from the second operation, but made no inquiries about breast reconstruction for a full year—and after making some initial inquiries, didn't decide to go ahead with the operations until the fall of 1986.

She explained why she waited, and then why she went ahead with the reconstruction:

"There was a period of time when I wasn't sure how long I was going to live. Every year I'd have to have a bone scan and a lung checkup to see if the cancer had spread, and I was very aware of the cancer. I was not making big decisions with long-term commitments. I couldn't do it. But then, after a while, after living with it, I slowly began to realize that I should be doing things that I really wanted to do, like buying a house," she said, gesturing around her living room. Another of those things involved a breast reconstruction.

"I can't speak for all women because all women have different reasons for what they do, either getting a reconstruction or not—and some reasons are big ones and some are little ones," she said.

"One big thing was that I wanted to look in a mirror and be happy about the way I looked. Not for anyone else, just for myself. I never really thought I had a spectacular body, but I was very comfortable with it. When I looked at myself I was very flat, very tight-skinned, you could see the bones in my chest. I feel good about myself, but there's a way you feel about your sexuality in the broadest sense, and I didn't feel right about that.

"Another thing was, every time I took a shower in the morning and looked in the mirror and saw my breasts gone, I was reminded that I had cancer. It's very depressing to have a daily reminder that you remain at risk, even when you're [otherwise] feeling pretty good.

"Reconstruction felt like a step toward getting on with my life. All right, I'd had cancer, but that's over with, let's get on with it," she said.

Some other things were less important, but nevertheless definite factors in her decision.

Since she had no breasts, she wore a prosthesis—but the prosthesis, she said, was hot in summer and cold in the winter.

"I hated to get up and put that cold thing on," she said. And it never looked right with her clothes. "Sometimes you just want to put on a T-shirt and forget about it."

While she was recovering from surgery, she had worked out with Encore, a support and exercise group for women who have had breast cancer. Cunningham came to speak, and she was impressed. She was further impressed when she saw a reconstruction he'd done of another woman's breasts. When she began to consider a reconstruction, she went to see him.

In September 1986, Cunningham implanted expanders under her chest muscles and gave her permanent implants two months later.

"It didn't hurt much. It felt more tight and sore, like you'd feel after too much exercise. You feel bruised, though you don't see any bruises," she said of the first operation. She missed four days' work, with a weekend in the middle, for a total of six days' recovery.

"When people talk about operations like this, they call them cosmetic, but that's a loaded word, because it seems to mean 'unnecessary.' I mean, you say, 'It's just like an arm or a leg,' and people say, 'Well, you really need an arm or a leg,' implying that you don't really need a breast. A breast is a part of a woman's body, and most women I know need them.

"Most of the women I met in Encore have the reconstruction for themselves. The ones who are married or have a significant other generally talk about those people as being very supportive. It's the women who need the breasts, not the men," she said.

Snapshot: Patients

His wife, Cunningham said, "keeps saying that the purpose of a face is to look normal. If it doesn't, it is diseased. The person is handicapped and needs treatment.

"There are more and more people who hold that view intuitively. When they feel their face has a problem, they look around for a way to repair it. The same thing for breasts or fat deposits and so on."

The explosive growth rate in the numbers of plastic surgeries of all kinds, both aesthetic and reconstructive, testifies to how many people are "looking around" for repairs. Suction lipectomies were experimental operations and almost unknown a decade ago. Now about 100,000 are done annually in the United States alone.

The rush for repairs has given too many people the idea that plastic surgeries, and especially rhinoplasties, are simple operations.

"That's a misconception," Cunningham said. "There can always be difficulties in surgery, and there can always be difficulties during the recovery."

If a person goes to an established, board-certified plastic surgeon for a common procedure like a rhinoplasty and shows no sign of either psychological or physical problems that would require extraordinary care, she will be seen at least twice before the procedure.

"The first thing I do is talk to the patient to see how clear her goals are. If she comes in for a rhinoplasty and says 'Well, I want to get rid of the bump and it's too wide,' that's pretty clear. That's the usual case, with most people. They know what the problem is.

"If somebody comes in and she's vaguely dissatisfied with her nose, that's more troublesome. It may take some time to determine whether surgery is indicated. Maybe she's just a little inarticulate. Or maybe she needs some other kind of help."

When he's decided a patient is an acceptable candidate for surgery, Cunningham places her in front of a mirror and stands beside her with a pointer. He asks her to point to each problem area and uses the pointer to make sure the two of them are in absolute agreement on what the patient sees as the problem.

Once the problem is clear, Cunningham outlines what can be done. In the case of a rhinoplasty, for example, that the top of the nose can be lowered and narrowed, that the wings can be reshaped, the nostrils made smaller and so on.

"Then we go away from the mirror and talk about the operation. How long it will take, how it's done, whether they'll be awake or asleep, what the pain will be like, what the bruising will be like. We talk about what can go wrong. That's an important part of the visit. Finally I take photographs, so I can study them here."

Cunningham's rhinoplasties are scheduled a minimum of two and a half to three months ahead of time. If the patient decides to go ahead with the operation, she will return about two weeks before the procedure for an examination.

"I walk her through the whole thing again—the mirror, how the operation works, what can go wrong."

Occasionally, a patient will come in with a photograph of a nose she's seen and likes, or that she feels will help explain to Cunningham what she is looking for. That also happens with breast-augmentation operations.

"Talking about breasts can be more difficult than talking about noses, because the problems with noses are often pretty apparent. The patient wants the bump taken off, and you agree that she'll look better with the bump taken off. With breast augmentations, though, you start talking about shape and size, and that's very hard to get to. You're talking about something the woman can see in her mind's eye, but is very hard to explain when you don't have a place to start."

There are times when Cunningham won't do what the patient wants—he won't, for example, make a nose or breasts too small.

"Patients are lay people, and they don't understand the effect of what they're asking for," he said. "In that case, you have to say that you won't do it. On the other hand, if I think a nose might look a little better one way, and the patient thinks it might look better another way, and she has a good, reasonable argument, then I have to go with her judgment. She's right, I'm not. She's the person who will be living with the nose. That's no problem."

Very rarely, a person will appear with a shopping list of changes that she wants done—rhinoplasties, augmentations, suction lipectomies.

"She goes back out the door with the list," Cunningham said. "I would feel uncomfortable working on somebody who has that kind of global dissatisfaction with her appearance. There are certain things that might go together. A face and a rhino, ears and nose, nose and chin. But if it's a case of reduce this, augment that, and suction the other, I won't do it. There's most likely some other problem there."

Between visits, Cunningham urges patients with questions to call him. Routine queries are often handled by his secretaries, Filus Tupa and LuAnne Zielinger.

"If somebody calls and says, 'Well, if I do this, will I have to stay in the hospital overnight?' Or 'What's the cost difference between going over to Samaritan or doing it at University?' Filus or LuAnne can help them. If it's 'Can you take off the bump and narrow down the tip and still leave me with some character?' then I'd handle that.

"It's absolutely critical to have an understanding with the patient, a relationship. The patient has to be comfortable with the idea of the surgery. Filus does a lot, helps with the administrative and personal details and the worries that somebody has when they're thinking about surgery. Sometimes a patient will want to talk to somebody besides the doctor. They see the doctor as this authoritative guy saying yeah, yeah, yeah, get the rhinoplasty, you'll look great, but the patient will come back to Filus and say, 'You don't really think I'm crazy to do this, do you?' "

When the talking is done, and the operation day arrives, Cunningham visits with the patient to make sure there haven't been any last-minute changes of mind. He also sees the patient at least twice after the work, even for the most complication-free procedures.

"In heart surgery, if the guy lives and the heart works, there's not much question that the surgeon did his job," Cunningham said. "It's a cloudier situation with plastic surgery. You can have a result that you think is great, but is not what the patient wants. If you're happy and she's not, that's not good.

"You've got to recognize that there are patients who'll always be dissatisfied. With the others, with the majority, you want them to leave happy. It's the best index of how you're doing."

Saving a Leg

HENRY WAS asleep on an operating table at St. Paul–Ramsey Medical Center under the beneficent influence of a single shot of sodium Pentothal. In less than a minute, he'd dropped from a sleepy semiconsciousness to the surgical level of anesthesia. Not even the grossest injuries would register with his brain, which was good: the surgery he was about to undergo was extensive and unconventional. A few years ago, it would have been flatly radical.

When Henry was unconscious, a drape covering his body was removed, exposing a long ugly burn. The burn ran from the tip of one hand, across his body, to the bottom of the opposite foot. The burn was irregular, but generally followed a narrow, crooked, "lightning bolt" pattern from top to bottom. Its color varied from a mottled tan to grayish-green. There were yellow-gray streaks around the edges of the most severely burned areas. The small toe on the burned foot was deep gray-green, like an old dry olive.

Henry, a Wisconsin strawberry farmer, had been knocking leaves and dirt out of a thirty-foot-long aluminum irrigation pipe when he was injured. Preoccupied with the blockage, he didn't realize how close he'd strayed to an overhead high-voltage power line. When the pipe touched the line, it was as though he'd been struck by lightning. As in many electrical accidents, the current followed body structures—muscles, nerves, and blood vessels—to the ground. The burns went deep.

"I really don't remember when the electricity hit me," Henry said the day before the operation. "It knocked me out. I came to shortly, but I guess I wasn't coherent. My son was with me—he was just burned a little, not bad—and he said some people at the greenhouse heard the fuss and came running over. I rose up and said, 'Can I help you?' and then sank back down again. They got an ambulance that took me into the hospital at Hayward [Wisconsin] and then a helicopter flew me down here to Ramsey."

The arm and chest burns, though extensive, could be treated without crippling effect. But a leg muscle, the one that controls the foot and covers the lower leg bone, had been literally cooked. This morning's operation would attempt to salvage the leg as a workable limb.

With Henry's body exposed, the nursing crew, under the general direction of the anesthesiologist and burn surgeon, began configuring it for surgery.

The anesthesiologist pushed a long breathing tube down Henry's throat, well into the windpipe, to protect against the possibility that he might vomit and then aspirate the vomit and choke. A rubber wedge went into the mouth beside the tube to keep his jaws open. His eyes were taped shut.

A nurse pulled out the arms of the operating table, and Henry's arms were stretched out in a crucifix position. One hand and arm, not involved in the operation, were wrapped in sterile blue towels to keep them warm.

Another nurse catheterized him, pushing a tube all the way up the penis to the bladder. The other end of the tube went to a plastic bottle under the operating table, which quickly accumulated a small puddle of urine. With the catheter operating, the nurse covered Henry's genitals with a sticky-edged plastic sheet to isolate them from the operating field.

("We usually do that, but it's not a matter of preserving modesty so much as getting everything out of the way and secured, and removing a possible source of contamination from the operating area," Cunningham explained later.)

A nurse washed portions of Henry's good leg with antiseptic soap. The leg had been shaved earlier that morning and would provide skin for grafts.

As the operating crew worked over Henry, a yawning nurse in plum-colored surgical scrubs ran into Cunningham in the hallway outside the OR and said, "Morning, Dr. Cunningham" through the yawn and Cunningham said, "How y' doing" and went straight on back to the locker room.

The men's staff locker room at St. Paul–Ramsey is old and battered, like part of an aging YMCA. Cunningham popped the combination lock on his locker, peeled down to boxer shorts and T-shirt, took a set of scrubs from a bin next to the locker-room door, and put them on. He slipped back into his loafers, covered them with disposable paper moccasins, and got a thin paper "shower cap" for his head.

Once uniformed in scrubs, hat, and moccasins, he stepped next door to the staff lounge, where Dr. Lynn Solem, head of the hospital burn unit, was chatting with a resident about the case.

Cunningham and Solem work together frequently. Though he runs the burn unit, Solem is also a general surgeon who can be found at odd hours of the day and night doing a variety of sometimes radical surgery on accident victims who have been everything *but* burned.

Henry was his patient. Solem was the person who decided that the leg might be saved by borrowing a muscle from another part of the body and plugging it into the leg (the operation called a "free flap"). It requires a specialist in microsurgery, and Solem asked Cunningham to do the work.

When Cunningham walked in they all said good morning,

and Cunningham popped open a can of juice that he'd brought in with him and then he said to Solem, "What are we going to do?"

Surgical talk tends to be laconic. The people involved have done preparatory examinations of the patient and have agreed on approaches and procedures. The conversations before the operation, and in the operating room, are carried on with a basis of much understood and agreed-upon information.

"Well, we want to look at that leg and see what we've got in there," Solem said. "I think we should be able to save it, but it'll take me an hour or so to get it all opened up and cleaned up so you can come in there, and we can decide what we want to do. . . . I mean there's either going to be stuff coming out of that joint or there won't be."

"Sounds good. I looked at it and it looks like there's a lot gone there, but it's mostly in that one line. . . ."

After a few more moments of general conversation, a nurse stuck her head in the door and said, "We're ready."

Cunningham wouldn't be needed immediately, so he went out to the operating suite's reception area to call his office for any last-minute changes of schedule. Solem got a surgical mask from a rack in the hallway, tied it on, spent five minutes washing his hands and arms in a scrub room, bumped the operating room door with his hip to get it open, and stepped inside.

The initial operating team included Solem; Dr. Jordan Sinow, a third-year surgical resident who would assist; Rose Schally, a certified surgical technician who would keep track of supplies and actually hand the necessary tools to the surgeons; an anesthesiologist and an anesthetist; two and sometimes three circulating nurses; and, on this particular day, a fourth-year medical student who would observe.

Schally was already robed in a sterile blue operating gown when Solem entered. She helped him into the sterile blue gown that goes over the scrub suit and into thin beige surgical gloves, and then helped Sinow, who followed Solem into the room.

Henry had been placed on the table to expose the operating field. A sheet taped to his upper chest acted like a tent to cover his face, blocking any view of his face from the operating table. Solem and Sinow took positions on the same side of the table while Schally stood opposite them, looking down at the now-anonymous collection of damaged meat, fat, bone, and tendon.

Solem started with a big scalpel. Without comment or ceremony, he began peeling away large chunks of skin and burned muscle on the lower leg, cutting down to living tissue. As he peeled away the flesh, he broke small veins and arteries, some of which were burned so badly they looked like dead twigs.

Other vessels were still viable, and began to bleed when they were severed. The bleeders were quickly cauterized by Sinow.

As more and more flesh was removed, baring the pearly white tendons of the leg, the leg began to look like the muscle-tendon transparencies found in high school biology books. Except for the gray burned flesh, even the colors were the same.

Blood began to accumulate in and around the wound as Solem got closer to good tissue. Sinow sopped it up with gauze towels and dropped the towels into a stainless-steel bucket by his feet. When the bucket got full, one of the circulating nurses would pull on thin rubber gloves (to isolate her from the blood) and, with the scrub tech, count out the towels in groups of five. "I count five towels," she said.

"I see five towels," said the scrub tech.

Only then were the towels disposed of: the operating team would lose track of nothing during the operation, to assure that nothing was left inside a wound when it was closed. There was not much chance of such a mistake in this case, but the routine is inflexible and is applied to all operations.

In forty-five minutes of steady work, Solem removed much of the skin and muscle from the front of Henry's lower leg. Cunningham came in and looked at it.

"No pus in that joint," he said.

"Naw, but there's been a lot of damage. Look at this," said Solem, pointing at a ragged complex of muscle around the ankle.

"This looks to be partially viable," said Cunningham. "Why don't we tangentially excise that and see if we can get back to something that's bleeding?"

"We've already lost a lot. I hate to lose any more than I have to. . . ."

"Yeah, but we can plug the flap in there, and go to, say, here. That will cover the ankle. . . . I guess the question is, will the tendon pus out? It's gonna be tough."

"If it was easy I'd get somebody else," said Solem, tongue-in-cheek, and the surgical tech snorted.

Solem went back to the leg, this time with scissors. After a few more minutes' work, he tossed them on the instruments tray and said, "That's enough. That's about enough."

Cunningham, who was wearing a mask but was not yet in a sterile gown, leaned close to the operating table but carefully avoided touching anything or anybody already sterile.

"Hell, if it doesn't work, he loses his leg and his rectus [muscle], and he would have lost his leg anyway. If it does work, he gets a leg he can step off on," said Cunningham. "Let's go ahead with it."

"Okay," said Solem, "let's do it."

The operation is complex.

Henry had suffered extensive muscle loss on the outside of the lower leg, just below the knee. That muscle, the tibialis anterior, controls the upward flexion of the foot. When that muscle and its related nerves are destroyed, the foot cannot be voluntarily flexed upward. And that is that. A muscle transplant won't help.

But the lower-leg muscle has another function besides flexing the foot. It covers, protects, and provides a living environment for the tendons that lie below it. Those tendons are attached to the lower-leg bones and are controlled by the muscles of the upper leg. It is those tendons, and those upper-leg muscles, that allow a person to step out.

(If you pick one leg up off the floor, and grip it with both hands, and then fold and extend the lower leg, you can feel the muscles of the upper leg at work. The folding and extending action is powered by the upper leg, but controlled through the tendons of the lower leg, which act like guy wires.)

If the lower-leg muscle is removed and not replaced, the tendons beneath it will wither and die. The whole lower leg will be useless. Cunningham proposed to save the leg by supplying a new "living environment" for it. He would do that by removing one of a pair of large muscles from Henry's abdomen and transplanting that muscle to the leg.

The transplant muscle is called the rectus. It is about as wide and thick as an average man's hand, and perhaps twice as long. It runs from the breastbone to the hipbone. It provides some protection for the body cavity, and also helps in the first few degrees of a sit-up. It can, however, be removed without serious functional loss. Because it's so big, and its blood supply is so well understood, it is a very handy muscle.

The muscle would be cut out of the abdomen and plugged into the leg. The operation called for a microsurgeon because an artery and vein from the transplanted muscle must be joined to an artery and vein in the leg. Since those blood vessels are perhaps one quarter of the diameter of a drinking straw, sewing them together requires highly delicate techniques performed under an operating microscope.

That work takes a specialist, somebody who does it with some frequency. Microsurgery is so delicate that it requires not only talent, but constant practice. Once a microsurgeon gets cranked up, he has to keep running. If his practice takes a different direction, say into heavier aesthetic surgery, he may have to stop the microsurgery altogether. It's not just something that can be done occasionally, as a sideline.

When Solem and Cunningham decided to go ahead with the operation, Cunningham left the operating table to scrub. He was tightly wound.

"You've got to get nerved up to do it because it's not very

tolerant of mistakes. One bad move and you turn the rectus into a three-thousand-dollar flank steak," he said as he scrubbed.

On another occasion, talking in his office, he said he was strongly drawn to microsurgery because of the challenge of doing something extremely difficult at which he was particularly good.

"About ninety-nine percent of the surgery done in America could be done by anybody with a reasonable mechanical ability, assuming that they are bright enough to understand the medicine in the first place. But there are some types of surgery that require such a complex understanding of the medium and such a complex understanding of your own talents and abilities that you just plain have to have a talent for it. If you don't have it, you can't do it," he said.

Now, as Cunningham scrubbed, Solem continued to do minor cleanup work on the upper leg, where the burn was not quite so bad. The portions of the leg already cleaned up—the exposed tissue in the lower leg, where the transplant would occur—were covered with damp towels to keep them moist. (The amount of garbage produced in the operation was substantial. A major operation, the nurses said, would produce eight to ten large plastic garbage bags full of gauze, towels, old bandages, drapes, and so on.)

Sinow, the surgical resident, had been assigned by Solem to remove Henry's small toe. He did that as Solem worked on the upper leg. The toe had been completely burned through by the electricity and was dead. The resident cut around the base of the toe, lifted it off the foot, and dropped it in a bottle held by the scrub tech. She handed it to the circulating nurse, saying, "Another piece for path [the pathology department]."

With the toe gone, Sinow began surgically reshaping the end of the foot. He trimmed down the bone that led to the small toe and trimmed some of the remaining skin and muscle. When he closed the wound, the foot had a smoother outside profile than if the toe had simply been lopped off.

By this time there was now a lot of blood around, on the towels and gauze pads and surgeons' operating gowns. A soft plastic bottle of blood, marked "A-POS" and colored the deep purple of cooked beets, dripped through a transparent tube into Henry's arm.

Every once in a while, Solem would question the anesthesiologist:

"What's his temp?"

"Ninety-eight point four."

"Looks like he's doing good."

"Oh, yeah, he's fine."

As Solem finished his cleanup, Cunningham bumped into the room, wearing a microsurgeon's version of bifocal glasses. In place of the bifocal inserts, these glasses have matching 6.5-power loupes protruding through the surface of the spectacle lenses like tiny twin telescopes.

"You okay?" he asked Solem.

"Yeah." Solem backed away from the table. Cunningham stepped up beside the patient, and he and the surgical tech loosened the drape that covered the patient's chest and pulled it away.

"Uh, knife," Cunningham said.

The tech handed him a scalpel, and with no further ado, Cunningham made a smooth but swift incision from Henry's breastbone to his pubic bone.

After the initial incision, several additional cuts were needed to get through a heavy layer of yellow fat to the underlying muscle. As Cunningham worked, Sinow, who had finished with the foot, hooked back the freshly cut tissue with retractors and sopped up the fresh blood.

Once down to muscle, Cunningham cauterized the bleeders. When he finished, there was almost no blood flowing in the large wound, but the room was filled with the smell of burned blood and fat.

With the bleeding stopped, Cunningham began dissecting the large rectus muscle from the overlying and underlying tissue. The muscle was held in place by webs of stringy white tissue called fascia (you can see it clearly on pieces of ham). It had to be cut carefully away, to minimize damage to other tissue. There were also blood vessels that went through the muscle into the fat layers and then to the skin, and those had to be cut and sealed with the cautery.

The pace was slow. Working alternately with a scalpel, scissors, and a cautery, Cunningham tried to dissect out the muscle as cleanly as possible. As he freed more and more of the muscle, the flap of abdominal skin and fat gaped open like a cardigan sweater.

Then a big step: Cunningham cut loose the bottom end of the muscle, near the pelvic bone. He stopped, bent forward, took the muscle in his hand, and frowned. Then he looked up at the resident.

"Look at this," he said, probing with his fingers and a small forceps. "It looks like they've been tied off, it looks like they're blocked." He gently lifted a bundle of what looked like desiccated worms, which were actually a vein and artery tied together with tissue.

Henry, it seemed, had had a hernia repaired several years earlier. Cunningham knew about that from Henry's medical history, and that operation should have had no effect on the rectus muscle. But it did. Cunningham now discovered that whoever had done the hernia repair "tied off the blood supply. . . . It looks like it was deliberate. . . . I don't know, I never saw anything like this before. This is not good."

Those were the blood vessels he had been planning to tie into the leg.

He went to the top of the muscle and found the vein-artery bundle there.

"This is the biggest superior pedicle I've ever seen; it must have compensated . . ."

He stopped working for a second and stood staring at the muscle in his hand, and then looked back again at the top of the muscle.

"I think we can go in with this," he said finally. He went back to snipping and cutting, but now there was a different air in the room: the operation was no longer difficult-but-routine. Now there was trouble, and Cunningham was moving into unknown territory.

Cunningham worked in near silence as he finished cutting the muscle from its supporting tissue and finally lifted it free from the patient's belly. Cunningham had now been working for two hours with intense concentration, his face dewy with perspiration under the sharp white operating lights. Just before noon, four hours after Henry was wheeled into the operating room and two hours after he started, Cunningham asked that the operating microscope be moved into place.

The microscope is a heavy instrument on its own stand, which fits over the end of the operating table. It is wrapped in its own surgeon's gown to keep its unsterile parts isolated from the table.

The scope has two separate eyepieces showing the same field. Cunningham stood on one side of the table, with Sinow opposite. Cunningham began dissecting a pair of blood vessels out of the leg tissue as Sinow watched. It was a lengthy job, and Cunningham stopped partway through, got a couple of Oreos stuffed under his mask, and took a hit of Coca-Cola through a straw.

Eventually, after a good deal more work, a pair of blood vessels, an artery and a vein, were located and freed for use. The idea was to tap into the leg artery and vein with the artery and vein from the rectus muscle, with right-angle joints. That would allow the leg artery to supply blood to the transplanted rectus and still maintain some blood flow to its usual muscle. The veins would take the blood back out.

When the leg vessels were ready, they were clamped and a small, careful incision was made in each of them. Just to be sure of the incision, the clamps were released and blood surged into the wound.

"That's veddy good," Cunningham said in a fake British accent as he reapplied the clamps. "Veddy, veddy good."

Tension had been building as he worked on the leg veins, and now it suddenly backed off and the whole operating-room crew began to relax. The rectus muscle had been freed from the chest and stomach, its veins and arteries identified, and Cunningham had found a good viable set of blood vessels in the leg that could be matched to the transplanted muscle.

"You know, all I can hear is this adenoidal breathing. Could we get a radio in here?" Cunningham asked cheerfully.

One of the circulating nurses said she thought there was a radio in another operating room not being used and asked an outside nurse to get it. The radio was wrapped in a plastic bag and brought into the room and tuned to Cunningham's favorite album-rock station.

"Jeez, that's the Doors," Cunningham said, looking up from the table. "Turn that up." Jim Morrison flooded into the room with "Riders on the Storm."

Cunningham went back to work, suturing the severed ends of the rectus muscle's blood vessels into the artery-vein pair from the leg. He never looked at his fingers on the needle holder, but only at knots forming in the field of the operating microscope. His fingers seemed barely to be moving; in the microscope field, the knots seemed to appear out of nowhere. The nylon thread used to do the sutures, size 9.0, was so fine and transparent that it couldn't be seen with the naked eye except when stretched directly through bright light. Then it glistened like a spider web or a scratch on a piece of colorless glass. As Cunningham made each knot, Sinow snipped the thread with a pair of scissors.

"Saw *Aida* last night," Sinow said, without looking up from the scope.

"Oh, yeah? Was it any good?"

"Oh, yeah, it was pretty good."

"I'm afraid opera's an acquired taste I haven't acquired," Cunningham said.

A few minutes later Cunningham finished the splice: "That should do it."

He made some final checks and then carefully removed the clips that had kept blood out of the vessels as he worked. Blood surged back into the vessels, and he watched a raw edge of the muscle. Nothing happened.

"It's not red enough," he said after a moment. He looked around the room. "We should be seeing more blood. The blood should be perfusing the muscle by now."

Sinow gently lifted the muscle to look at an edge where it had been cut free from the chest.

"We're seeing a little around here," he said.

"Should be a lot more than that," Cunningham said. He sounded angry. "If we don't get enough blood in there, the muscle will die."

Then: "Let's wait a few minutes."

He stepped back from the table and looked around, and the tension in the room cranked up again.

"Could you turn the radio down a notch?" he asked a circulating nurse, though the radio was not playing very loud. He looked back down at the muscle. "It's not working. We're going to have to take it down."

He explained: "We might not be getting enough blood pressure through there with that right-angle joint. We have to take it head-on. The tissue fed by that artery can get enough blood from other sources to compensate, if it has to. . . ." He waited another minute, but there was no change in the muscle. "Let's take it down," he said.

He and Sinow went back to the microscope, reclamped the artery and vein, and tore out all the careful stitches. Then Cunningham severed the incoming blood vessels and restitched them head-to-head to the blood vessels in the transplant muscle. If that join did not work, the muscle would not be viable, and the patient would lose his leg. He would also lose the stomach muscle—it would become, as Cunningham had said earlier, a three-thousand-dollar flank steak.

The tension cranked up again as the last few stitches went in. The operating room was absolutely silent.

Cunningham finished, looked around, and said, "Here we go," and removed the clamps. Nothing happened for a second, two seconds, then blood began to pour from the cut edges of the muscle. The sides of the muscle turned a bright, shiny pink. "Here we go up here," said Sinow.

Cunningham: "Looking good, that's looking good."

They watched for a few minutes, then Cunningham backed away from the table, obviously pleased.

"Listen," he said, "leave it like that for a minute. I gotta go tap a kidney, and then we'll come back and see how it's working."

Though Cunningham had interviewed and examined Henry before the operation, he never once saw the man's face in the operating room.

"That's the best way to do it," he said later. "I don't want to have to deal with a personality. I don't want to have to deal with the idea that I'm working on this person who has all kinds of hopes and expectations. I have enough to deal with right there on the table. I can't worry about anything else.

"If you're working on somebody who you have a personal relationship with, and you keep thinking, Jeez, I can't screw this up, I can't ruin my friend's life by losing the leg, then you're more likely to screw up. You've got to go in there and do the best you can. Fix it. And if it doesn't work and the guy loses his leg, you can't brood over it or you'll start freezing up. And you will brood over it if you start thinking of patients as friends and trying to make real relationships with them on the table. Once they get on the table they're just a patient. That's the only way you can deal with it."

When Cunningham returned to the operating room, the muscle was bright pink, the splice apparently working fine. Cunningham rerobed and finished the operation, a relatively routine matter of tacking the muscle in place and covering it with skin grafts. He left most of the work to Sinow.

"I'll tell you, for a minute there I thought we had a problem with those [clogged vessels at the bottom of the muscle]. It worked out," Cunningham told Solem, the burn surgeon, who had come back into the room.

"Ah, we knew you'd save it, Bruce," said the surgical tech, who was cleaning up the instruments.

And he had. A few months after the operation, a newspaper ran photos of Henry walking around on the roof of his north-woods home after a blizzard, shoveling off the snow.

Snapshot: Big Moves

A few weeks after the free-flap operation on Henry, Cunningham sat on his office couch in an expansive mood, joking with his secretary Filus, and talking about plastic surgery. Henry's operation came up, not only because it was a tough one, but because the rectus free-flap is, in some ways, Cunningham's baby. The talk of Henry's flap led to a rambling commentary on the nature of American medical care.

"I did my master's thesis on the thing [rectus flap]," he said. "Nobody much was using that muscle, and we had a feeling that it could be pretty handy. The research showed you could take it [out of the abdomen] without losing a lot of function.

"Anyway, I did background work on it, went down to the cadaver lab, went down to the postmortem area, and dissected out a bunch of them, measured them, measured the [blood] vessel size. We figured it would work, so we did a couple. It worked fine. We took it on the road, to conferences and so on. Now it's used in most of the major microsurgery centers," he said.

It takes a certain kind of personality to make big surgical moves. It takes nerve, determination, and a bit of showmanship. It also helps to be in the right place at the right time.

"The environment is important," Cunningham said. "Us guys at the university are lucky, because we're expected to experiment and do research, and we get support for it. You need support, because if you do experimental work long enough, you're going to screw up. With support, you'll keep going; if you screw up and everybody jumps on you, after a while, you'll start playing it safe all the time. Then you won't be the guy who makes the big moves."

Cunningham once did an operation on a man who had had both

heels destroyed by frostbite, leaving him unable to walk. Because lower-leg prosthetics are so good, some doctors might have been tempted to go ahead and amputate the legs. Others might have tried two cross-leg flaps. In that operation, the legs are pinned together, and a muscle from one leg is attached to the heel of the foot on the opposite leg. When blood vessels from the foot grow into the flap, the flap is severed from the leg, and a new heel built with the replanted tissue. Then the whole process is repeated on the other side.

"It'd take forever and be very expensive," Cunningham said. So he did a free flap. He took a chunk of muscle, attached it to both heels at the same time, pinned the legs together for three weeks, and, when the blood vessels from the feet had grown into the flap, the flap was cut in half and the man had two new heels.

"The thing is, there are always problems when it hasn't been done before, and you're in a place that won't give you support for doing something new. Then you might say, 'Forget it, let's stay with the standard therapy,' which is to take the legs off."

There are many hospitals, Cunningham said, where a patient like Henry would have lost his leg, and needlessly.

"Yeah, the doc would look at it and say, 'Let's get on with it, he's going to lose it,' because he never heard of the [free flap] operation, or he wouldn't have the facilities to do it, or because of insurance problems or any number of things.

"One of the problems the medical profession is facing right now is that the way [Medicare and insurance] transactions are handled, smaller hospitals have a strong financial incentive to hold onto a case, even if it's beyond their capability to take care of it.

"I'm not saying that if they have an obvious and outrageous trauma that needs a Room Ten [a St. Paul trauma-specialty team] that they're going to take him back in their OR and start working on him; but there are all these borderline cases, where the tendency is to say, 'Well, let's hang on for maybe a couple of days, we can probably handle this.'

"So you get these people calling the burn unit and they say, 'We have this guy with a fifty-percent burn, and gee, I can't remember, what's the best fluid management for them?' You can't say, 'Listen, turkey, buy a book or send them in here,' so one of our guys will say, 'Okay, this is what we do. . . .'

"And then the guy says, 'Oh, gee thanks, listen, you're still using Silvadine on them, that's the dressing you're using now, right?' Basically, some guy is getting a lesson in acute burn management over the telephone and some patient is paying for it.

"In the past, these guys [doctors] would say, 'Jeez, I'm not taking care of this, send him in to the Cities,' and that would be that. But now their hospital administrators are leaning on them to hang onto cases awhile, give it a try. So now you've got more and more cases where the patient might get dinked around for a couple of weeks, and then get sent to us, and by then, well, like [Henry's] leg, if that had happened, all the tendons would be dried out and infected, and then it's too late.

"That Wisconsin hospital did just right. They looked at him and said, 'The hell with it, send him to the Cities,' and put him on a helicopter. There are places, lots of places, maybe even most places, where he would have lost the leg.

"And you know, getting him down here still might not have helped if we didn't have some people who were willing to let you take a shot at new things. If you sat down and thought about it, you could come up with a lot of reasons why a free flap on [Henry] was stupid. First of all, we take a valuable piece of meat out of the guy's belly and stick it on his leg after we know the guy's had electrical burns. So what if it had gotten infected and fallen off and been a disaster? Somebody could have come along and said, 'You moron, electrical current is transmitted along blood vessels [and might have damaged them enough to make them useless], everybody knows that, you should have known you couldn't hook them up.' You could find all kinds of reasons for not doing it, playing safe.

"It wasn't that long ago, thirty years, forty years, when heart bypasses were crazy, and not long ago heart transplants were nuts, and kidney transplants and liver transplants.

"Sometimes I worry that we're losing the environment that

201

lets us do those kinds of things. People say, 'Okay, so you can save the guy's life by transplanting his heart, so what? He's just another guy, and he's going to die sooner or later anyway, and probably sooner because his heart's so bad, why spend so many of society's dollars on fixing him up? Let him go, and spend the dollars on somebody who's got a while to live.'

"You hear that more and more. But that kind of attitude is basically antiprogress, antiresearch. If the transplanters keep doing work, someday the operations will be routine and affordable and lots of people will have them, just like bypasses today. But they won't get there without all the big expensive research operations we're doing now.

"You need the environment to make the big moves. I hope we keep it."

A New Thumb

A FREE flap, like the one done on Henry, is impressive. At the same time, it is essentially passive. It protects whatever function the leg still has, but doesn't improve it.

More advanced and more difficult than an ordinary free flap is the creation of a working, functioning body part. At 8:00 A.M. the week before Christmas in an operating room at St. Paul–Ramsey Medical Center, Cunningham was about to start the most difficult operation he does.

He was tense, "nerved up," as he calls it, getting everything just right. He repeatedly checked the patient as the anesthesia was administered, checked the tools, supervised the tuning of the radio. When he was finished, classic album rock bounced softly off the gray-green tiled walls and blue-speckled terrazzo floors. A jumble of monitoring equipment, glowing with green and yellow and red digits, fed a dozen tubes and wires into what looked like a pile of blue laundry on the operating table.

A child lay under the piles of sterile blue sheets, buried except for his right arm and left foot. Even his head was covered: he breathed through a respirator, each breath registering on an electronic monitor. His eyes were taped shut.

Cunningham hunched over the child's perfectly formed, waxy-pale left foot. He wiggled around in the swivel chair a bit, getting settled, poked among a selection of scalpels laid out on the tool tray, and finally picked one up. Holding the diminutive knife as though it were an artist's pen, he made a series of sketching motions that left behind short, shallow incisions at the top of the arch.

"There's the vein," he said, probing through the webs of skin, fat, and connective tissue. "The artery will be deeper."

The work was slow. The critical elements involved—an artery, a vein, and two nerves—are delicate and easily damaged.

Snipping and searching with tiny scissors, Cunningham isolated the two blood vessels from surrounding tissues. The artery posed an immediate problem.

"Boy, it's small," Cunningham said. "It's the smallest I've seen. The last kid I did wasn't as big as this one, and his artery was bigger. I don't know if this is going to work."

Cunningham crossed his gloved hands on his sterile robe and peered down at the incision. A minute passed. He sat silent and unmoving, contemplating the artery which lay in the incision like a purplish, desiccated worm. Then he picked up the scalpel and opened the incision a bit farther.

"It should work," he said finally. "We can look at it some more, but it should work."

Cunningham commonly does two or three or even four operations in a single day. On this day there would be only one, and it would take the whole day, eleven hours, from dark winter morning to dark winter evening, working over the child. There was nothing wrong with the boy's foot. His hand was another matter.

A year earlier, the nine-year-old had been helping split firewood with a power log-splitter. There was an accident, and his hand was caught and smashed. The splitter crushed his ring finger, cut diagonally through his hand below the middle and index fingers, and chopped through his thumb above the bottom joint.

The kid got to Cunningham a few hours after the accident. Cunningham replanted the index and middle fingers, but the smashed ring finger and the top part of the thumb were pulped. They were completely unsalvageable.

Now, a year after the accident, in an excruciatingly difficult piece of microsurgery, Cunningham would remove the second toe from the boy's left foot and use it to build a new thumb. Functionally, he would not miss the toe. Cunningham said that after his foot healed, the missing toe would not even be especially noticeable when the boy was walking barefoot.

"We're going with this [left-foot] toe because you get better sensation on this side," Cunningham said, indicating the side of the second toe that faces the big toe. "When we replant it [as a thumb], that side will be against his hand, and he'll get better sensation, better pinch."

The child, buried beneath the sterile blue sheets, was oblivious to the team working around him in the cool odorless air of the operating room.

"We keep him covered to keep him warm," said the nurse-anesthetist, who sat at the boy's head. "Kids have a lot of body surface area for their size and they can lose heat fast." The temperature monitor showed the boy's body at 99.2°, only a few tenths above normal. "That's just fine," the anesthetist said.

In addition to Cunningham and the anesthetist, the surgical team included two surgical technicians and a circulating nurse.

A fifth person, a third-year surgical resident, would assist in the latter part of the operation.

Cunningham wore the usual operating gear—surgical mask and cap, thin rubber gloves, and knee-length sterile paper gown. He was also wearing his loupe-spectacles, with the two magnifying scopes protruding through the lenses like miniature cannons.

And only a few minutes into the operation, he was worried. That artery was awfully small.

The artery, which takes blood into the toe, and the vein, which takes it out, had to be dissected from several inches above the toe. The long blood vessels would be needed to reach down the hand from the transplant site, on the stump of the thumb, to connect with blood vessels coming into the hand.

The blood vessels of the foot are hidden in bundles of muscle and connective tissue. Dissecting them from that tissue is a long, tedious job, and it must be done perfectly the first time—a mistake could irreparably damage the delicate vessels.

As operations go, this one was boring for all of the operating crew but Cunningham: he sat hunched over the foot for four long hours, using a variety of small tools to free the blood vessels and nerves and to identify two tendons that would also be used in the reconstruction. The hunched position is an occupational hazard, often leading to a troublesome back. The tension doesn't help, either.

The biggest problem Cunningham faced in this operation involved the artery. There was some doubt whether it was big enough to carry enough blood to keep the transplanted toe tissue alive, even if it could be cleanly dissected from the foot. Although the artery was the main blood supply, several smaller blood vessels also fed into the toe. When the toe was severed from the foot and reattached to the hand as a thumb, the smaller vessels would be gone—and the artery would be the sole source of blood.

In addition, the join itself would tend to reduce the amount of blood that could flow through the vessel, at least until it healed. If the vessel proved too small to deliver the needed quantity of blood, the transplant would die.

With the size of the artery questionable, it was critical that it be extracted without damage. Doing that is roughly equivalent to picking up a fistful of cooked spaghetti, squeezing it into a lump, and then dissecting out one soft strand as it runs through the center of the clump, without breaking or even nicking it— and, at the same time, doing the least possible damage to the lump itself. It takes time. Cunningham sat and picked and picked and picked.

By noon, the blood vessels had been freed from surrounding tissue, although they remained intact, carrying blood to the toe.

206

The nerves had also been isolated. Cunningham had identified and mentally tagged the tendons that bend the toe; they would be attached to the remnant thumb tendons.

The actual amputation of the toe went quickly. It was removed from the foot at the lowest joint. The ball joint at the end of the metatarsal, the long bone coming down the top of the foot, gleamed in the raw tissue of the wound like a pearly white marble. The blood vessels, though exposed, were left intact so that they could continue supplying blood to the toe as long as possible.

"Let's get his legs down," Cunningham said, pushing back in his operating chair and standing up. The boy was lying on his back, with the legs bent sharply at the knees. Most of the blood flow to the leg had been cut with an automated tourniquet, similar to the tourniquets nurses wrap around patients' arms when they're taking blood-pressure readings.

With help from a surgical tech, Cunningham removed the pads supporting the boy's legs. The pressure on the tourniquet was dropped. The toe remained waxy pale for a few moments, then slowly began to turn pink.

"That's definitely good," Cunningham said with evident relief. "The artery will support the toe by itself. There still might be a problem when we reattach, but it looks good."

Cunningham covered the toe with gauze pads soaked in saline solution and stretched. He had done ten previous toe-to-thumb transplants. All were successful.

"With this operation you have all the problems you get with a replant, with the additional problems you get with taking the toe off and matching the sizes [of toe to thumb] and locating the blood vessels and the nerves.

"When you're reimplanting, you're working with damaged tissue and you just do the best you can. With this thing, there's all the planning and thinking and the work of getting [the toe] off while doing the least damage, which is the hardest part of the operation—and then you have to do the whole replant when you finally get it off.

"It's an operation with tremendous benefits. You give the guy half his hand back. In evaluations of physical impairments, loss of a thumb is considered to be fully the loss of half a hand."

Cunningham didn't mention it, but it's clear that an operation like this is also a rehearsal for a straight transplant, moving a body part from a brain-dead donor to a living patient. With a reconstruction using the patient's own tissue, however, there are no problems with immune reactions. The tissue can be transplanted without threat of immune rejection. Solving the immune problem—and Cunningham believes the solution is near, and perhaps even has arrived—would mean that straight transplants could be done immediately: the surgical techniques are already in use.

The assisting resident entered the room as Cunningham finished with the toe and moved to the boy's hand, which was laid out on a wing of the operating table.

With the resident opposite him, Cunningham cut into the wrist just below the thumb joint, where the blood vessels would be spliced. The incoming vein and the artery were found, isolated, and covered with saline-soaked pads.

The surgeons then trimmed the covering tissue off the stump of the thumb, exposing the raw bone. Cunningham tunneled under the skin of the thumb from the exposed stump to the incision on the wrist where the vein and the artery were exposed. Later, the artery and vein would be carried back from the transplant, through the tunnel to the connection to the incoming blood vessels of the arm.

With the hand ready, Cunningham moved back to the foot. After making some measurements, he quickly severed the toe's blood vessels and brought the toe up to the hand.

The basic join between toe and thumb was made by matching raw bone ends while orienting the toe so that when flexed, it would oppose the rest of the hand. The toe was then sewn tightly to the stump of the thumb with wire sutures. Eventually, the bones would grow together.

With the basic join done, Cunningham located and spliced the thumb stump tendons to the equivalent tendons in the toe.

"You want the scope now?" asked the circulating nurse.

"Yep, bring it up."

The binocular operating microscope was rolled into place over the hand. While Cunningham worked it into place, the resident began closing the foot wound.

Splicing the nerves took Cunningham twenty minutes of work under the scope.

"The way it works is that a new nerve ending [from the stump of the thumb] will grow right up the nerves in the toe," Cunningham said. "When it's all done, he ought to have good sensation all through the thumb."

After Cunningham finished with the nerves, he used a loop of suture thread to lead the toe's exposed blood vessels through the tunnel of skin to the incision on the wrist. Through the microscope, the wound showed a red background of fibrous tissue, spotted with small areas of yellowish fat, white connective tissue and nerves, and the dark line of the artery. Cunningham clipped the arm artery to stop blood flow and then severed it.

The resident finished the foot, moved to a seat across the table wing from Cunningham, and peered into the second eyepiece. He and Cunningham began manipulating the blood vessels.

The artery was about the diameter of a pine needle on a Christmas tree. Cunningham put eight stitches around the artery and tied each with a square knot. Then he did the same with the vein. The needle he used was smaller and thinner than an eyelash, and the monofilament nylon thread was so thin that it was invisible to the naked eye, except when it glistened in the beam of light from the microscope.

There were indications that it would work, but the ultimate test of its viability would come only when the feeder artery was unclipped and blood was allowed to flow through the splice. Given the small size of the artery, Cunningham feared that the slice itself would reduce blood flow enough to kill the toe.

The test would come now.

Cunningham peered through the microscope, making a last check of the splice; nodded, leaned away from the scope, and carefully removed the clips on the feeder artery and its paired vein.

For a moment, nothing happened. The artery in the lower opening, where the splice was, began to beat with a pulse as the blood flowed through. Above the join, the thumb still looked pale as death.

If it was going to work, Cunningham said, "it should pink up pretty quickly."

"It looks pinker to me," the resident said hopefully.

"You think so?"

A surgical tech crowded in a bit and decided that the toe definitely looked pinker.

"Okay, look at this," Cunningham said, indicating an area of raw tissue. "We're getting some blood here . . . and we're getting some out of that vein."

And suddenly, more blood flowed into the wound, indicating that the toe—the thumb now—had circulation. And a moment later, the skin on the toe blushed a light, pretty pink.

"All right," Cunningham said hoarsely. "It's not as pink as it should be, but it's getting there."

The rest was cleanup—more supporting sutures, bandaging, and a splint to hold the bone join rigid until it healed.

When the healing is completed, Cunningham said, the toe functions quite well as a thumb. It even looks pretty good.

"It looks a lot better than you'd think. The toe—the thumb—gets bigger with lots of use, and starts to look like a regular thumb, kind of, except that it has an extra joint. But it's not the kind of thing you really notice unless you look. The same thing with that missing toe. When we close it, we close the gap [between the big and third toes] so you'd never notice that a toe was missing unless you counted them. It's just not the kind of thing you notice around the swimming pool. So the aesthetic quality is damn good."

The toe-to-thumb operation, Cunningham said later, was among the toughest he did.

"It takes such sustained concentration. You spend hours dissecting that toe out and there's no such thing as making a bad move. A bad move and you've just indulged in a very expensive waste of time. And then after you get it done [the toe removed], you've got to put it back on. Boy, I'm glad that's over."

The operation, from start to finish, took just over eleven hours.

"That artery was so small," Cunningham said, the weariness showing in his voice. "I don't even like to think about it."

Snapshot: Other Operations

Cunningham does operations of one sort or another almost every weekday. Most are routine: skin grafts, the removal of small skin cancers, or scar revisions—making a large ugly scar into a small neat one.

He does not do harelip or cleft-palate repairs, because those are done by his wife and a third partner. In addition, his wife does highly technical penis reconstruction surgery in cooperation with a urologist.

Nor does Cunningham do the complicated cranial-facial surgery that attempts to reconstruct congenitally misshapen heads of children. "That's interesting work, but it's also a complicated and technical specialty. I just don't have the background or training for it. You can only go so many ways, and I went with the microsurgery."

Some of his operations are distinctly peculiar.

In one case, a large brain tumor was growing through a woman's skull. The neurosurgeons who would remove the tumor faced the problem of re-covering the brain: since the skin and bone both would be removed, the woman would be left with a large hole in her skull. Cunningham was called in and did what in burn cases would be a routine scalp expansion. The expansion provided the skin to cover the wound when the tumor was eventually removed. It was interesting because as far as he knows, it had not been done before quite like that, but it was not a serious technical challenge.

Every year he does one or two nose reconstructions, building a new nose from skin taken from the patient's forehead. It's one of the oldest operations done by plastic surgeons—its history stretches back several hundred years—but is also somewhat unsatisfactory.

"What the patient winds up with is not a particularly aesthetically pleasing nose, but it's about one hundred times better than walking around with a hole in your face," Cunningham said.

Of all the operations he's done in the past two years, one stands out for him, and another for the author of this book, and for dramatically different reasons. Cunningham's favorite operation provided some of the happiest results he's ever had: "it might be my best piece of work." In the author's favorite operating-room scene, nothing happened at all.

Cunningham's best piece of work began with a small, ugly farm incident.

A thirteen-year-old boy was feeding a horse on his uncle's farm. Suddenly the horse reached out with its teeth, grabbed the boy's lower lip, and tore away the lip and the fleshy part of his chin. The boy's screams brought quick help. The torn tissue, a flap of flesh between two and three inches in diameter, was packed in snow. The boy was taken to St. Paul–Ramsey Medical Center.

The wound was grotesque—there was simply no covering over the lower part of the boy's face. From the teeth down, he looked like a living, bloody skull.

"When I came in, the lip was on ice. They took him off to get him ready for the operation, and I sat up there in the operating room looking at the lip, trying to find a couple of blood vessels that I could reattach to keep it alive, to get some blood pumped in there. I knew where there was an artery—there's an artery right along the edge of the vermilion [the pink part of the lip] and I eventually found it. The veins were so small there just wasn't any sign of one. I just couldn't find anything. There are no named veins in the area.

"But I had that artery, and [an assisting surgeon] brought him in, and we hooked it up. And I took the clamp off, and the goddamned thing turned pink! There was blood going through there. It was just about the most thrilling moment of my surgical career.

"I mean, if this didn't work, this kid has a huge problem. It would have taken him years, years, to get a mangled-up mass of tissue on his lower lip that would never have looked like a lip but that would keep him from drooling all over himself. He would be out of school, he would be an invalid, he couldn't go out in public, his life would be shattered. But if it works, he just kind of keeps to his normal schedule.

"And when I took off that clip, the goddamned thing turned pink. I started to think we might be able to save it. So then, I had the blood going in, but I needed a way to get it back out. We had the nurses turn his head down, which causes the veins to fill with blood. We found one tiny little vein on the lip and paired that up with the flap on the other side, and we got blood going out."

Cunningham still wasn't sure the lip would live. It was almost two weeks before he became confident of success: by then, small capillaries had established themselves across the wound lines, providing another source of blood.

In the succeeding weeks, he got a bonus he never expected. Nerves from the boy's face grew down into the torn tissue, giving him almost full control over his lip muscle. Cunningham showed him off one day in a clinic checkup.

"Okay, watch this. Do this," Cunningham prompted, pursing his lips.

The boy managed a partial pursing. Cunningham was delighted.

"When we first put the lip on, there was no movement at all, and he couldn't feel a thing. Saliva would pool in the fold of his lower lip, but he couldn't feel it, and he'd be drooling without knowing it.

"Now he has feeling all the way around the chin area; you can see the way he purses his lips. The nerves from the upper face must have grown down into the chin area. It's pretty amazing, and it probably wouldn't have happened if he wasn't so young. If this happened to you or me, at our age, we'd be out of luck.

"As it is, this [recovery] violates all the rules, that he should be able to get this much motion and control and sensation."

He turned to the boy. "Smile for us?"

The boy smiled. Cunningham beamed.

. . .

Several weeks after showing off the lip repair, Cunningham walked into an operating room ready to work. He was about to create the author's favorite OR incident. The patient was asleep, and the nurses had finished removing the thick layer of bandages on his right leg. A resident was standing by to assist.

"He Kawasakied himself," Cunningham said. (Kawasakied is surgeon-talk for an injury in a motorcycle accident. One emergency-room doctor referred offhandedly to motorcycles as donorcycles, since they contribute so many young, healthy, brain-dead bodies to the transplant wards.)

In this case, the bike slipped out from under the biker, and together they skidded down a gravel road until they hit a mailbox. The mailbox took a cube-shaped chunk of muscle and bone out of the front part of the biker's lower left leg. The bone shattered with the impact. It was now held in alignment with a stainless-steel brace that was screwed through the skin and muscle directly into the bone.

The case belonged to the hospital's orthopedic surgeons. Cunningham had been called in as a consultant, to move some of the remaining lower-leg muscle to cover exposed bone and tendon in the cube-shaped hole.

He never got to it.

"Boy," he said, "this guy doesn't smell so good." He bent fully over at the waist, put his nose next to the exposed wound, and took a long sniff. Not satisfied, he continued to sniff up and down the leg. There was an odor of fleshly corruption.

"That's not fresh; there's some junk in there," he said.

"He didn't smell too good when they brought him in—the wraps we took off him were ripe," said a nurse.

"Open that [garbage] sack," he told a nurse. She pulled a plastic bag out of a waste container and opened it. "Smell that? Smell that," Cunningham ordered the author. "Stick your head in there. Can you smell that?"

I stuck my head in the bag and sniffed. The impact was . . . was equivalent to climbing out of your car on a hot summer day, walking back to the three-days-dead cat on the road, kneeling down, and inhaling the aroma.

"Yeah, I got it now," I said, trying to suppress a gag. The nurse watched in amusement.

"I think we have trouble," said Cunningham. He went off to scrub, came back, got into the sterile gown and gloves, and began to work over the wound. He stopped occasionally to sniff, and after a few minutes, shook his head.

"This needs more time. It's got to be cleaned up better than this," he said, stripping off his gloves and canceling the operation. "No fun and games today, boys and girls."

The decision was an important one.

"You can't let yourself be pressured by the social situation. Here you are, all ready to go, and somebody else has said his patient is ready and wants you to come in and do some work, and the nurses and tech are all ready, and you have to say, 'Nope.'

"If I put a flap [muscle transplant] over dead tissue, it won't take. Then I've not only failed to help the guy, you've damaged him further. There's nothing wrong with using your nose to figure out things. You've got to use everything you've got."

A week later, the wound was in better shape and he did the procedure. Six weeks later, the biker admitted that the leg worked so well that he was riding his Harley again.

But it was an interesting moment, there in the operating room, when Cunningham called off the operation. In a surgical suite with several millions of dollars' worth of diagnostic and moni-toring gear, it all came down to a couple of noses. Not something you'll see on TV.

Transplant

THE TRANSPLANT is waiting. Cunningham can do it. The surgical techniques are proven. The chemicals are available.

He would remove a hand from a brain-dead donor and transplant it to an amputee. The recipient's nerves would grow into the donor hand. The bones, blood vessels, and tendons would fuse. Eventually, the recipient would develop sensation and grip.

"He won't play the piano, but his hand will be a hundred times better than any prosthesis," Cunningham said.

The essential barriers to the transplant are not technical, but political and ethical.

Cunningham began considering the technical problems and philosophical justifications of a hand transplant several years ago as he was developing his skills as a microsurgeon.

"Amputees tend to be people who work with their hands. If there's an explosion or a fire or their hands are crushed or caught in farm machinery, the accident often involves both hands," Cunningham said.

The loss of both hands, particularly to people who earn their living with their hands, is essentially the loss of meaningful life, Cunningham argues. He believes that for selected people, a double amputation justifies the use of the most innovative surgical techniques to return one or both hands.

(There are also accidents that involve both feet, but Cunningham is not nearly as interested in a foot transplant as he is in a hand transplant.

"Prosthetics for foot amputees are remarkably good. You wouldn't gain enough with a transplant to make it worthwhile," he said. Prosthetics for hand amputees, however, simply can't do many of the things we routinely expect hands to do.)

Even as Cunningham completed the structural studies and mastered the surgical techniques that would allow him to do the transplant, there remained serious medical barriers to the operation.

The human body has a self-defense mechanism called the immune system. In ways not fully understood, it identifies and attempts to eliminate invading or foreign organisms.

Unfortunately, the system is mindless: it identifies even life-saving transplants as foreign and rejects them. Rejection is a major cause of failure in heart, liver, kidney, and pancreas transplants.

The immune system can be suppressed with drugs. But there are drawbacks. The drugs can be directly dangerous, poisoning and damaging vital organs. And they can be indirectly dangerous: since they suppress the body's defensive mechanisms, they open the way to infections and diseases, including certain types of cancer.

The risks are sometimes clearly justified.

"Everybody agrees," Cunningham said, "that it's okay to suppress the immune system when a person's life is in jeopardy, when he needs a new heart or liver. If the worst thing happens, and the patient dies [from effects of the immunosuppressants], he's no worse off than if he'd died in the first place. On the other hand, if the treatment works, you've saved a life.

"For some people, the corollary to that argument is that you don't suppress the immune system unless it will save a life. A hand transplant isn't lifesaving. It may improve the quality of life, it may allow a person to work again, but it's not essential to life itself."

Even as he refined the skills necessary to do a hand transplant and became convinced that a hand transplant was surgically possible, Cunningham essentially agreed with the conservative position on immunosuppressant drugs. They were too dangerous to use in non-life-threatening cases.

His first hand-transplant proposal to the university suggested that a transplant be attempted only under very special conditions. He asked permission to work on a person who was already immunosuppressed. Like a diabetic.

Some background:

Among the candidates for lifesaving organ transplants are severe diabetics. Diabetics suffer from a disease of the pancreas, which is a soft, nondescript, five- or six-inch-long organ that huddles behind the stomach. Hormones secreted by the pancreas help the body regulate blood sugar levels. Failure of the pancreas can lead to a variety of difficulties, including, in severe cases, coma and death.

Animal hormones, extracted from beef and pork pancreases, can be used by most diabetics to regulate blood sugar. For a few people, though, animal-hormone therapy does not work. Faced with a life-threatening condition, and with no other effective options, they become candidates for pancreas transplants.

It also happens that diabetes is frequently accompanied by vascular disease, manifested in problems with blood circulation. As the blood vessels choke down in the arms and legs, gangrene may occur. Eventually, it may be necessary to amputate hands and feet or entire limbs.

It should be possible, Cunningham thought, to find a pancreas-transplant patient who had also lost a hand. Since that person would already be immunosuppressed (to support the transplanted pancreas), he could receive a hand transplant with no further immunosuppression.

The idea was interesting, but there were problems.

A diabetic who is ill enough to require a pancreas transplant is not an ideal candidate for any kind of nonemergency surgery. It is also possible that the persistent vascular disease that caused the amputation in the first place would jeopardize the viability of the transplant.

From a research point of view, the diabetes and the treatment of the diabetes might obscure the processes of the hand transplant. Of course, if the hand worked as expected, if the nerves grew back to the fingers, if the recipient developed sensation and grip, some key research questions would be answered.

The last possibility was tantalizing enough that Cunningham submitted a formal proposal to the University of Minnesota's Human Experimentation Committee. After some negotiation, he was told to go ahead. But only if he could find a volunteer recipient already immunosuppressed.

That, as it happened, was not easy. One woman appeared to be a possibility, but she was terribly weak and very ill. Cunningham feared that she simply could not support a transplant.

As they waited for another candidate, Cunningham and his research associates began to change their position on the use of immunosuppressant drugs.

"When we used [early immunosuppressant drugs] there was pretty good reason to worry about their effects. But then a new drug, cyclosporine, came along. The established dosages are so low that the danger of adverse side effects seems minimal and acceptable.

"Say we take an individual who is not immunosuppressed, and suppress him, and do the transplant. Sometime later he shows signs of getting in trouble with the cyclosporine, some kind of adverse side effect. So we reduce the dosages even more, or eliminate them altogether. If the patient loses the hand, well, he's no worse off. And he may have gotten years of improved quality of life from it. . . .

"It seems almost too obvious, but it's very important that the hand is on the outside of the body. You can monitor it, you can see it, you can deal with every little thing that comes along. It's not like a heart or a liver, where you really don't know from day to day exactly what's happening. With a heart, you can be in bad trouble before you know anything has gone wrong. With the hand, you can look at it every day. You can see what the trouble is."

By the end of 1986, Cunningham had decided to push the new approach, based on the arguments that cyclosporine was safe enough to justify the attempt, that any complications could be carefully watched, and that even if a transplant failed, and the hand had to be removed, the recipient would be no worse off than he had been originally.

And, he would argue, all this information would be presented to the patient before the start of the work. The patient would know the risks and the possible benefits. Let the patient decide, Cunningham said.

The politics of research surgery are vastly unlike the practice of surgery itself: they move neither quickly nor surely.

Before he could do the hand transplant, Cunningham needed the approval of two University of Minnesota committees: the Ethics Committee and the Human Experimentation Committee.

The committees were not rubber stamps. The moral, ethical, and legal questions they juggled were not of the angels-on-a-pin variety, but the harsh realities of late-twentieth-century medicine: of life and death and endless lawsuits.

Missteps made in human experimentation could have frightening consequences, and not just for the experimenter and his subject. A whiff of looseness could damage the university's entire transplant program—its pride and joy—and slow progress in collateral fields of medicine.

"They have to be conservative," Cunningham said. "The problems are too complicated just to say to anybody, 'What the hell, go ahead.' But we've been conservative, too, about this whole transplant project, and now it's about time. We're almost ready, and we ought to make the move."

There was also an unspoken consideration behind the politics.

It might be called the Fame Conundrum, and it was stated with brutal clarity by a scientist in a completely different field: "To be wrong is bad," he said. "To be second is nothing."

A successful first hand transplant could add substantial luster to any surgeon's reputation. And that is the question that haunts ethics committees. Might not a surgeon be willing to do a marginal operation on the chance that it would succeed and confer upon him substantial public celebrity, rather than labor in relative obscurity?

There had been accusations in other places, at other times, about top medical reputations—unsavory matters at best. And since a university research hospital is a large place, and not everybody knows everybody else, how to tell whether any particular doctor is a serious researcher or a simple opportunist?

The committee routines—the necessity of defending your proposals—are designed to deal with that problem. Which makes the routine no less frustrating for those going through it.

So Cunningham wrote the letters, lined up the testimony, and waited. Would the project be approved?

"I dunno," he said one day at lunch as he sat behind a bowl of parsnip-and-black-mushroom soup at a French restaurant. "They won't buy the whole thing. They never do. There'll be restrictions, for sure. But I'm hopeful. The big guy [Dr. John Najarian, head of the university's surgery department and a leading national proponent of transplant therapy] has written a strong letter and I've sent a strong letter. If they just let us in, just an inch. Just let us do it that first time. *Just that first time.*"

Six months later, Cunningham had his approval to immunosuppress a patient and transplant a hand. He also had another problem. While he was fighting his proposals through the Ethics and Human Experimentation committees, he attended a plastic surgeons' conference in which hand transplants were discussed.

There were substantial differences of opinion about whether a transplant would be functional. Worse, there was a challenge to some of the research on which Cunningham had based his transplant proposals. The work had been done in Canada, using baboons, and the results had been promising. Later, parallel research at an American institution had come up with less-promising results.

"We're going to have to look at it," Cunningham said. "I don't know. I still think we're ninety percent good, but it's something we have to check out."

The review took the rest of 1987, but by early 1988, Cunningham and his researchers had decided that more animal research would be pointless.

"We're close. We're going to have some possible candidates come in for examinations and tests," he said in January 1988.

He thinks about the transplant quite often—if the medical world accepts the idea that immunosuppressants can effectively and ethically be used in nonlifesaving situations, the impact could be considerable.

One day in the operating room, he was working over a little girl whose body, head, and arms had been terribly scarred by fire. She had virtually no hair, and one hand had been so badly burned at the time of the accident that doctors were forced to amputate it. She would live with the scarring and the baldness forever. Unless . . .

"Do you realize what we could do if we could immunosuppress this kid?" Cunningham said, suddenly looking up from the table, his blood-dappled gloves hovering over the anesthetized girl's head. "If we could immunosuppress her to give her a hand, there wouldn't be any reason not to give her hair, too. We could really fix her up. God, if you could find some way to deal with the immune system, you could really do miracles, you know?"

It's that kind of talk that will get you somewhere.

Statistics I

Aesthetic plastic surgery is the fastest-growing specialty in medicine. The following statistics illustrate the numbers of surgeries for two recent years, the growth in the numbers, and the number of surgeries performed on males. Although males have always been in the minority for all plastic-surgery procedures save one—hair transplants—the numbers of men seeking other aesthetic surgeries is rapidly increasing. Currently, among those aesthetic plastic surgeries done, about 16 percent of the patients are male. The following statistics are taken from the most recent survey of board-certified plastic physicians done by the American Society of Plastic and Reconstructive Surgeons.

Procedure	1984	1986	% Change	On Males (1986)	Male % (1986)
Abdominoplasty (tummy tuck)	20,900	32,340	+55%	2,264	7%
Blepharoplasty (eyelid lift)	73,900	84,690	+15%	15,244	18%

Procedure	1984	1986	% Change	On Males (1986)	Male % (1986)
Breast enhancement	95,000	93,540	−2%	—	—
Breast reconstruction	98,800	57,270	−42%	—	—
Breast reduction	37,700	48,600	+29%	—	—
Chemical peel	16,200	15,600	−4%	624	4%
Dermabrasion	23,500	26,280	+12%	7,096	27%
Forehead lift	—	15,900	—	1,590	10%
Hair transplant	4,500	2,790	−38%	2,650	95%
Mastopexy (breast reshaping)	16,200	17,160	+6%	—	—
Mentoplasty (chin augmentation)	17,500	15,330	−12%	2,759	18%
Otoplasty (ear revision)	13,200	14,880	+13%	6,547	44%
Rhinoplasty (nose reshaping)	70,500	82,830	+17%	20,558	25%
Rhytidectomy (facelift)	54,400	66,930	+23%	6,693	10%
Suction lipectomy (suction-assisted fat removal)	55,900	99,330	+78%	5,966	6%

Statistics II

The cost of plastic surgery varies widely from surgeon to surgeon, from hospital to hospital, from city to city, across regions, and from one nation to the next. The cost of particular procedures may also vary depending on the amount of work to be done and the complexity of the operation. The cost of a breast reconstruction, for example, may depend on whether one breast or two are to be reconstructed. Mentoplasties, or chin augmentations, are often done in conjunction with rhinoplasties—nose jobs. The combination of the two surgeries may cost sharply less than the two surgeries priced and done separately. The following price list, then, is simply a general guide. It is based on fees charged by board-certified plastic surgeons, according to surveys done by the Society of Plastic and Reconstructive Surgeons.

Procedure	Fee
Abdominoplasty (tummy tuck)	$2,000 to $6,000
Blepharoplasty (eyelid lift)	$1,000 to $4,000

Procedure	Fee
Breast enhancement	$1,800 to $4,000
Breast reconstruction	$1,000 to $7,000
Breast reduction	$2,000 to $5,000
Chemical peel	$250 to $3,000
Dermabrasion	$250 to $2,500
Forehead lift	$1,000 to $4,000
Hair transplant	$250 to $4,000
Mastopexy (breast reshaping)	$1,500 to $5,000
Mentoplasty (chin augmentation)	$250 to $3,000
Otoplasty (ear revision)	$1,000 to $3,500
Rhinoplasty (nose reshaping)	$1,500 to $6,000
Rhytidectomy (facelift)	$2,000 to $10,000
Suction lipectomy (suction-assisted fat removal)	$500 to $4,000

Acknowledgments

Many people helped collect information for this book, and I am particularly grateful to a number of patients—in the book, they are all given pseudonyms—who allowed me to observe their operations and who cheerfully answered what sometimes were intensely personal questions.

Bruce Cunningham showed immense patience and courtesy in allowing me to follow his work and in answering, honestly and without hesitation, hundreds of questions that at times must have struck him as hopelessly naïve.

Several medical and professional people are mentioned in the text, all under their real names, and I am grateful for their help. Dozens of other medical and professional people at St. Paul–Ramsey Medical Center, the University of Minnesota Hospitals, and at Samaritan Hospital in St. Paul also were unstinting of their help. I thank them one and all. Their professionalism and humanity were wonders to behold.

And finally, I would like to acknowledge a considerable debt to Filus Tupa, Cunningham's secretary, who kept me up-to-date on his operations, helped make appointments with his patients, and suggested source works that I might want to read as background.

Index